Environmental and Ecological Statistics

Series Editor
Ganapati P. Patil

For further volumes:
http://www.springer.com/series/7506

Environmental and Ecological Statistics

Series Editors

G.P. Patil
Distinguished Professor of Mathematical Statistics
Director, Center for Statistical Ecology and Environmental Statistics
Editor-in-Chief, Environmental and Ecological Statistics
The Pennsylvania State University

Timothy G. Gregoire
J.P. Weyerhaeuser, Jr. Professor of Forest Management
School of Forestry and Environmental Studies
Yale University

Andrew B. Lawson
Division of Biostatistics & Epidemiology
Medical University of South Carolina

Barry D. Nussbaum, D.Sc.
Chief Statistician
U.S. Environmental Protection Agency

The Springer series **Environmental and Ecological Statistics** is devoted to the cross-disciplinary subject area of environmental and ecological statistics discussing important topics and themes in statistical ecology, environmental statistics, and relevant risk analysis. Emphasis is focused on applied mathematical statistics, statistical methodology, data interpretation and improvement for future use, with a view to advance statistics for environment, ecology, and environmental health, and to advance environmental theory and practice using valid statistics.

Each volume in the **Environmental and Ecological Statistics** series is based on the appropriateness of the statistical methodology to the particular environmental and ecological problem area, within the context of contemporary environmental issues and the associated statistical tools, concepts, and methods.

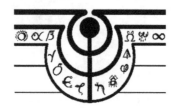

Wayne L. Myers · Ganapati P. Patil

Multivariate Methods of Representing Relations in R for Prioritization Purposes

Selective Scaling, Comparative Clustering, Collective Criteria and Sequenced Sets

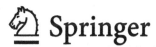 Springer

Wayne L. Myers, Ph.D.
Penn State Institutes of Energy
and Environment
Pennsylvania State University
University Park, PA, USA

Ganapati P. Patil, Ph.D., D.Sc.
Center for Statistical Ecology
and Environmental Statistics
Department of Statistics
Pennsylvania State University
University Park, PA, USA

ISBN 978-1-4899-9028-0   ISBN 978-1-4614-3122-0 (eBook)
DOI 10.1007/978-1-4614-3122-0
Springer New York Dordrecht Heidelberg London

Printed on acid-free paper

Springer is part of Springer Science+Business Media (www.springer.com)

We dedicate this work to a transformative spirit of cooperation and collaboration that we have seen spreading across statistical sciences in recent years. The **R** *software system is a monumental example of such spirit, both in its open access and its fostering of collaborative contributions through the CRAN compendium of extensions. While* **R** *is an outstanding example, it is by no means the only such effort. The Python programming language is of a similar order of open sharing, as is also the Open Geospatial Consortium (OGC). Each of us has endeavored to personally promote such cooperation and collaboration: Prof. Patil through the Center for Statistical Ecology and Environmental Statistics in the Department of Statistics at Penn State University, and Prof. Myers through the Penn State Institutes for Energy and Environment. Working with each other through decades of our careers has enhanced both of our efforts toward making joint work more than the sum of the parts. We carry the collaboration forward after transitioning to emeritus status.*

Preface

This monograph is multivariate, multiperspective, and multipurpose. We intend to be innovatively integrative through statistical synthesis. Innovation requires capacity to operate in ways that are not ordinary, which means that conventional computations and generic graphics will not meet the needs of an adaptive approach. Flexible formulation and special schematics are essential elements that must be manageable and economical.

We find that the computational context of the **R** statistical software system is quite convenient for meeting these needs. **R** is easily available without charge and extensively augmented by CRAN contributions. Compared to other language-like software systems, **R** gives the user high-level commands while allowing many modifications on an optional basis along with capability for custom composition. **R** is keyboard and keyword controlled, however, as opposed to being mostly mouse-a-matic. Consequently, some learning and experimentation are required to proceed proficiently. A purpose of practicality is thus to be enable Rs of those who are interested enough to delve deeply into data and pursue practice. To encourage this degree of dedication, we have a didactic dataset that threads through all but a couple of the chapters. This demonstrative dataset is sufficiently small to be entered entirely by a patient person in a single session, but extensive enough to provide practice by selecting several subsets. An auxiliary of appendices is provided for preliminary practice with **R**.

A philosophical purpose is to accomplish some attitude adjustment with regard to analytical alternatives that tend to be conceived as competing. We encourage shifting the concept of *competition* to *complementary* insofar as appropriateness of assumptions may allow. We promote what we call "comparadigms" of comparative analysis whereby insight is gained from differences that emerge by varying views, such as scalings and statistical strategies. The underlying question here is *when does a (statistical) difference make a difference (that is evident or suggestive)*? The extra effort of traveling alternate routes to an intended end can either offer insights or be comfortingly confirmatory.

We further transmute *competing* into *coupling* through what we will call *data distillation* to distinguish it from other monikers, such as data mining. Packaged protocols of statistical systems typically all have the same starting point of the basic data table (matrix). We will often do differently by feeding forward the results of one analysis into another analysis as a chain of informational condensation. Many analytical activities act as filters that mute minor messages and amplify aspects of major messages. We thus have a progressive process of obtaining overtones and portraying prominent patterns. Retaining results from intermediate operations allows for stepping back to add interpretive undertones that may also carry important implications.

Another point of perspective lies in remembering that data are dualistic as interplay between observational instances and values of variates. There are variations in the view with addition or deletion of cases, and likewise for variates. This is clarified by considering each case to be a sort of signaling device, and the variates to be transmissive channels for conveying content. A crucial question in probing for patterns is whether certain subsets of the case devices are projecting peculiar/particular patterns on some of the channel variates. Such dual decomposition of data is the essence of data distillation.

Interwoven throughout this thematic tapestry is a primary purpose of promoting partial prioritization. This problem is pervasive in modern society from environment to economics. Complete prioritization is often quite contentious, but picking the best of the better and the worst of the worse will often suffice to allocate available resources and alleviate partisan paralysis. Since combinatorial computations are often involved in prioritization, preliminary partitioning into similar sets can rapidly reduce the computational concerns. Therefore, clusters of cases and characterizing collectives can be crucial. While objectivity is essential for circumventing conflicts, it is also essential not to exclude expertise. Transparency is likewise a critical concern, for which easily deciphered displays are especially effective. We have endeavored to present the particulars in a manner that is accessible and acceptable to a spectrum of professional practitioners as well statistical specialists.

University Park, PA, USA   Wayne L. Myers
                                                                                    Ganapati P. Patil

Acknowledgments

We gratefully acknowledge the United States National Science Foundation Project 0307010 for Digital Governance and Hotspot Geoinformatics of Detection and Prioritization for its support of parts of research that underlie this approach. We likewise express gratitude to Penn State University for its continuing accommodation of our work as emeritus professors; both in the Department of Statistics and Penn State Institutes of Energy and Environment as well as the School of Forest Resources.

We give gratitude beyond measure to our wives Faith Myers and Lalita Patil for their supportive patience, and also extend thanks to other members of our families. Many colleagues and collaborators are deeply appreciated, even if not named individually.

About the Authors

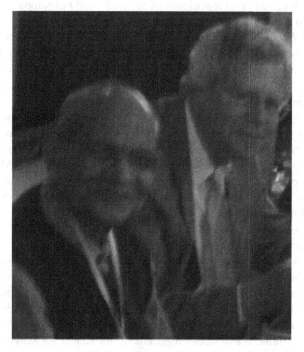

Dr. Wayne L. Myers is Professor Emeritus of Forest Biometrics, The Pennsylvania State University. He specializes in landscape analysis using geographic information systems (GIS) and remote sensing in conjunction with multivariate approaches to analysis and prioritization. He is a Certified Forester under the auspices of the Society of American Foresters, an Emeritus Member of the American Society of Photo-grammetry and Remote Sensing, and a 40-year member of the American Statistical Association. He has pursued a transdisciplinary career path seeking synthesis among spheres of science and service. This began with a Bachelor of Science in Forestry at the University of Michigan (1964) including research assistant work in forest economics and biological aide for the US Forest Service on mountain pine beetle in Ogden, Utah. Membership in Phi Beta Kappa reflected the liberal arts component of his interests, Phi Sigma reflected biology, and Xi Sigma Pi reflected forestry. Then ensued a Master of Forestry degree in Forest Ecology at the University of Michigan (1965), during which he was a teaching fellow in forest tree physiology and garnered the Phi Sigma Society graduate award for achievement in biological sciences. His Ph.D. work at the University of Michigan (1967) focused on Forest Entomology and the quantitative aspects of populations under a National Science Foundation project, being completed while employed as a research scientist in forest entomology at the Forest Research Laboratory, Ontario Region of Canada Department of Forestry where he subsequently shifted focus as Regional Biometrician.

He joined the faculty of Michigan State University in the Department of Forestry at the age of 26 with responsibility for the disciplinary field of forest inventory. At MSU, he was received into the societies of Sigma Xi and Phi Kappa Phi. With colleagues at MSU, he conducted seminal studies of remote sensing from satellite platforms when NASA launched its initial Earth Resource Technology Satellites which subsequently evolved into the Landsat Program. These initial interdisciplinary studies were continued under NASA's Skylab program. Another of his focus areas at MSU was the development of general purpose computer software in the FORTRAN language for multivariate analysis.

He was delegated to the forestry faculty program of USDA Forest Service in 1974, working with the Region 6 Office, Timber Management Division in Portland, Oregon on continuous forest inventory. In 1976, he was given a foreign assignment from MSU as consultant in the Brazilian Federal University of Vicosa, Minas Gerais to help develop research and teaching in forest biometry. During a sabbatical leave from MSU in 1976, he undertook authorship of a book on Survey Methods for Ecosystem Management to provide an early interdisciplinary perspective on inventory of natural resources. This effort reached fruition in 1980 with publication by Wiley-Interscience.

He moved to the Pennsylvania State University in 1978 with the School of Forest Resources, where he also assumed responsibility for faculty level management of the Experimental Forest along with expanding research interests to include water resources. At PSU, he joined the faculties of the Intercollege Graduate Degree Programs in both Ecology and Operations Research. A collaboration with Prof. G. P. Patil was also initiated as a faculty associate for the Center for Statistical Ecology and Environmental Statistics. Soon after arriving at PSU, he accepted an interagency personnel agreement (IPA) assignment with USDA Forest Service, State and Private Forestry, Northeastern Area, Broomall, Pennsylvania concerned with the analysis of information needs and information management in comprehensive statewide forest planning. This led into the pioneering area of GIS for which he developed software systems and explored applications in the context of the PSU Experimental Forest. The combination of work in remote sensing and spatial information systems engendered a 1984 joint appointment as Codirector of the Office for Remote Sensing of Earth Resources in the Environmental Resources Research Institute at PSU. In

1986, he participated in a team visit to India organized by Prof. G. P. Patil, and then in early 1987 obtained a travel grant for 2 months' work in Taiwan, India, and Malaysia. In turn, this led to a 2-year expatriot assignment as Forestry Advisor to USAID/India Mission under Joint Career Corps contract between PSU and USAID during 1988 and 1989. The JCC term in India included work on social forestry, natural resource sustainability, biodiversity, water resources, and GIS; including preparation of the USAID tropical forestry and biodiversity assessment for India. In India, work also raised an interest in computer-based expert systems and artificial intelligence.

After returning to PSU from India, international work and biodiversity continued to be an integral part of interests and activities. This encompassed three summer research fellowships in Malaysia at Forest Research Institute Malaysia (FRIM) and KUSTEM University in Terengganu; additional work in India with a watershed initiative at Moolhi Jaitha College in Jalgaon, India; collaborative outreach in Poland and Ukraine; and research workshops and collaborations in Norway, Switzerland, Italy, and Indonesia among others. Biodiversity became a central issue as coleader of the Pennsylvania GAP Analysis assessment of vertebrate habitats in conjunction with the larger National GAP Analysis Program. Habitat concerns continued to be prominent in a landscape level ecological classification system developed in cooperation with the Pennsylvania Bureau of Forestry.

In the first decade of the new millennium, Prof. Myers served as Assistant Director for Graduate Studies in School of Forest Resources at PSU and as Director of the Office for Remote Sensing and Spatial Information Resources in the Penn State Institutes of Energy and Environment. He has received the Twentieth Century Distinguished Service Award in Statistical Ecology, Edward Bellis Award in Ecology at PSU, Boggess Award of American Water Resources Association, Community of Teaching Excellence Award at PSU, and Outstanding Faculty Award in School of Forest Resources at PSU. He has authorship in several books and/or parts of books along with numerous research articles. He retired from the teaching faculty of PSU in June 2009 with the status of Emeritus Professor. He continues working in research, writing, and workshops both domestically and abroad.

Dr. G.P. Patil is a Distinguished Professor of Mathematical and Environmental Statistics Emeritus in the Department of Statistics at the Pennsylvania State University, and is a former Visiting Professor of Biostatistics at Harvard University in the Harvard School of Public Health.

He has a Ph.D. in Mathematics, D.Sc. in Statistics, one Honorary Degree in Biological Sciences, and another Honorary Degree in Letters. He is a Fellow of American Statistical Association, Fellow of American Association of Advancement of Science, Fellow of Institute of Mathematical Statistics, and Elected Member of the International Statistical Institute, Founder Fellow of National Institute of Ecology and Indian Society for Medical Statistics.

He has been a founder of Statistical Ecology Section of Ecological Society of America, a founder of Statistics and Environment Section of American Statistical Association, and a founder of the International Society for Risk Analysis,

International Society for EcoHealth, Society for Syndromic Surveillance and Digital Government Society of North America. He is founding editor-in-chief of the international journal, Environmental and Ecological Statistics and founding director of the Penn State Center for Statistical Ecology and Environmental Statistics.

Dr. Patil has published 30 volumes and 300 research papers. He has received several distinguished awards which include: Distinguished Statistical Ecologist Award of the International Association for ecology, Distinguished Achievement Medal for Statistics and the Environment of the American Statistical Association, Best Paper Award of the American Fisheries Society, and the Best Paper Award of the American Water Resources Association.

He was a member of the UNEP Science Advisory Panel with Nobel Laureate Mario Molina for the UNEP Division of Environmental Assessment and Early Warning. He recently served on the NSF Panel for Homeland Security and Geographic Information Systems. He has been on the Science Advisory Board of the Spatial Accuracy Symposia. In the recent past, he has served on the EPA Science Advisory Board Regional Vulnerability Assessment Panel and chaired a UNEP Expert Panel for Human Environment Index.

Dr. Patil has been recently principal investigator of a large NSF project on digital governance and surveillance hotspot geoinformatics for monitoring, etiology, early warning, and sustainable development. This has involved upper level set scan based geospatial and spatiotemporal hotspot detection and partial order theory-based multicriteria ranking and prioritization with several national and international live case studies.

Contents

Chapter 1
Motivation and Computation

Our primary perspective lies with practical procedures for strategic screening and partial/progressive prioritization when there are multiple measures containing comparative criteria for substantial sets of informational instances. Computational considerations impose constraints on combinatorial comparisons, and perception of patterns for visual verification helps to cope with complexity. The open source data analysis system called **R**© (R Development Core Team 2008) is well suited for this coupling of computation and cognition. We seek secondarily to provide a portal into the realms of **R** through exposition by example. For continuity of comparison, we concentrate on a dataset of cellular conservation characteristics for the State of Pennsylvania (Myers et al. 2000). This has been a favorite dataset for us in illustrating innovative analytical approaches since it allows us to incorporate spatial proximity into the comparative context. This dataset is shown in Appendix 1, and provides the present point of departure. The **R** software can be downloaded via the **R**-project Web site http://www.r-project.org making it readily available to all. Appendices 2–5 offer a springboard for those who are unacquainted with **R** consisting of introductory learning exercises that have served as the basis for workshops to introduce **R** protocols.

We configure what might be called *comparadigms*. We collect data on instances of interest in terms of multiple observable properties through some protocol(s) of quantification to obtain a matrix (table) of data. By means of analytical methods we then compare several properties on the individual instances and compare the properties across instances to obtain prominent patterns. The information available for comparison is inherently dualistic—it arises jointly from the choice of instances on which to observe properties and from choice of properties to observe on instances. An instance can be considered informally as a sort of signaling device for monitoring a complex contextual environment and the properties (or indicators) as channels through which signaling is being conducted. Interest lies in analyzing the outputs of the several such devices to determine clarity of signals and characterize complexity regarding comparative status of the environments being monitored.

Many or even most analytical approaches provide ways of filtering the outputs to enhance clarity and determine collective modes of operation with regard to signaling.

W.L. Myers and G.P. Patil, *Multivariate Methods of Representing Relations in R for Prioritization Purposes*, Environmental and Ecological Statistics 6, DOI 10.1007/978-1-4614-3122-0_1, © Springer Science+Business Media, LLC 2012

We are most interested in *prominent patterns* or *major messages* that emerge from the data domains; and, in this sense, *data distillation* might be an appropriate adjunct to the jargon of *data mining*. Underlying our approach is intent to promulgate precedence of preference among instances for partial and/or progressive prioritization while lending logic and logistics to public portrayal of a prioritization process. The imperatives are often to target the best of the best as prime prospects or the worst of the worst as critical cases, leaving the mixed messages for later etiological investigation of interactions. Note that our use of the term *precedence* in relation to preference among instances is not to be confused with the so-called precedence-type statistical tests for comparison of treatments with a control which focus on the order of occurrence for outcomes (Balakrishnan and Ng 2009).

Our approach is unconventional in asserting that multiple views have greater prospect of revealing prominent patterns than single views, so we couple what are often seen as competing methodologies while looking for commonalities and contrasts. We suggest analytical sequences whereby the results of one analysis are fed into another analysis instead of starting over directly from the data. Each analysis in such a sequence becomes a sort of filter that feeds forward amplified aspects of major messages while muting more minor messages. We do not insist on showing statistical significance as a prerequisite for probing possibilities. We do, however, use distributional models as frames of reference. In the course of these pursuits, we endeavor to demonstrate how each analytical activity serves as a lens for learning.

Since terminology can be a source of confusion, it should be addressed carefully as the need arises, and some such is appropriate at the outset. The term *case* is shorter than the term *instance* and, although it has several other meanings, is not likely to cause confusion when used as a substitute for *an **individual** instance* herein. A specific set of cases having some commonality is called a *collective*. Analysis can be conducted at the level of either case or collective, with collective constructs being useful for controlling complexities of computation. In addition to using the terms *case* or *collective* instead of instance, we use the term *variate* for a property as quantified by a specified protocol with these quantities **varying** from case to case. It is this case-to-case variation that is of primary interest, since complete uniformity of quantity across cases becomes only a composite characterization rather than a comparative characteristic. When variates satisfy special strictures, they will be considered as investigative *indicators*. We thus consider a *multivariate data matrix* that comprises n cases or collectives of cases as rows and p variates or investigative indicators as columns along with a leading column of IDs.

Plan of Presentation

We begin by delving directly into our data domain and its conservation context followed by a briefing on basic building blocks of architecture in **R** (Venables et al. 2005; Hogan 2010). After cursory consideration of command context for **R**, we pursue parsimony in a simplifying sequence of scalings for variates. Starting with original observations, statistical standardization serves to suppress differences due to units of measure. Relative ranking further removes distributional differences, leaving only ordinal aspects of analysis. This threefold suite of scalings makes an ideal introductory platform for applying special scaling schematics in **R**, such as parallel boxplots and "pairs" plots of lattice graphics (Verzani 2005; Crawley 2007; Horton and Kleinman 2011). We then move to complexities of covariances and correlations among multiple measures as reflections of their relationships and redundancies. This leads to rotational rescaling regimes and abstract autonomous axes as virtual variates "packaged" in terms of principal component analysis (PCA) and disposable dimensions.

Creating collectives by clustering can circumvent computational constraints, cope with complexity, and simplify schematics. Dealing with disparities as distances is common in clustering, and there are many methodological modalities and depictions as dendrograms. Combinatorial keys to clusters can be inferred from classification and regression trees (CART). Conflicting clusters from alternative approaches can be reconciled by comparative contingency. Contingent clusters can be cast comparatively in low dimensional distance domains called principal coordinates (PCO) by methods of multidimensional scaling that concentrate on capturing neighborness with minimal structural stress that would induce distortion. Skeletal structures of networked neighbors can serve to show sensitivities to scaling scenarios.

Prioritization perspectives progress from collectives to cases. Rating regimes for ascribing advantage and perceptual precedence plots furnish a framework connected to concepts of partial ordering (Brüggemann and Patil 2011). Subordination schematics and representative ranks become combinatorial constructs for condensing criteria and ORDIT ordering for sequencing of sets. Coupling of comparatives and salient scaling promote partial prioritization. Cases of clarity lie in convergent corners of coupled comparatives, whereas complexity and confounding are characteristic of a mixed middle. Median mismatches are functional features for investigating interplay of indicators. Rank rods, end extents, and distal data diagnostics reveal candidate cases for remediation and retention whereby a particular criterion is substantially degrading overall status or elevating otherwise inferior status. Complementary cases can be chosen in progressive prioritization by revising ranks so that advantage accrues only if a candidate has one or more ranks that are better than those found among previous picks. Landscape linkages can contribute to configuring criteria where selections are spatially specific. Constellations of criteria can be considered in confronting complex contexts.

Although matrix mechanisms underlie much of the methodology, they receive minimal mention in the main parts of the presentation. So that the matrix function facilities of **R** are not neglected, however, some of the earlier exposition is revisited and extended in a mechanistic matrix mode. The focus here is on virtual variates obtained by rotational transformation and inverted accordingly as may be appropriate. The purview that we present provides a pathway for pursuing particulars of partial order and systematic selection from sequences of sets.

Data Domain

The setting for our data domain is the State (Commonwealth) of Pennsylvania in the USA partitioned by a tessellation/zonation into 211 hexagonal cells with each cell encompassing 635 km². The hexagonal cells have been numbered as part of a North American grid whereby the numbers increase along northeast to southwest sequences of cells. Thus, there are breaks in the numbering for Pennsylvania as the sequences of cells enter and leave the state. The geographic arrangement of cells and numbering is shown in Fig. 1.1.

As a further frame of reference, Pennsylvania is situated in northeastern USA with New York State on its northern (upper) border and the northwestern corner jutting up to Lake Erie. The topographic character of the state is shown by virtual hill-shading in Fig. 1.2. This reveals the overall geologic and physiographic character of the state, with predominance of the sandstone-based Appalachian Plateaus in the west and north where weathering of rock produces rather coarse-textured and infertile soils that do not support extensive agriculture involving row crops. Eons of erosion in the Appalachian Plateaus have created deeply cut river valleys and rugged terrain in the uplands with extensive forest that may be quite fragmented in some subregions.

To the east and south of the Appalachian Plateaus region is the strongly folded area known as Ridge and Valley which curves from south-central to northeast in the state. Here, the hard rock and thin soils of the ridges are mostly covered by forest,

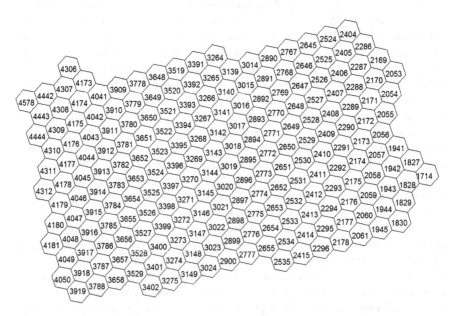

Fig. 1.1 Hexagonal cells and cell numbering for Pennsylvania in northeastern USA

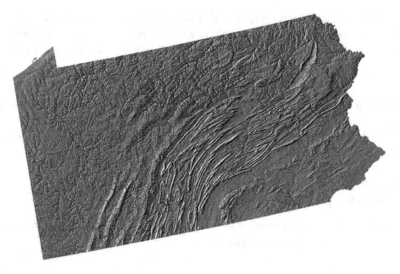

Fig. 1.2 Hill-shading depiction of topographic character of Pennsylvania

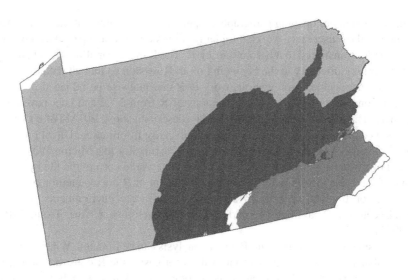

Fig. 1.3 Major physiographic/ecoregional areas of Pennsylvania

whereas the valleys are primarily agricultural and/or urban/suburban. The Ridge and Valley is flanked to the southeast by the broad agricultural corridor of the Great Valley. The southeastern (lower right) sector is a more subdued plateau called the Piedmont which has quite fertile soils with extensive agriculture and urbanization leaving only remnant patches of forests. Figure 1.3 shows the general physiographic/ecoregional partitioning.

Given this general biogeography, rather pronounced differences in the character of the landscape are to be anticipated along with differing capacities to provide habitat for fauna and flora. In this context, the hexagon data has six variates as follows.

BirdSp is the number of bird species for which there is potential habitat in the hexagon.

MamlSp is the number of mammal species with potential habitat in the hexagon.

ElevSD is standard deviation of an elevation grid in hexagon (topographic complexity).

PctFor is percent of hexagon with forest.

Pct1FPch is percent of hexagon in one contiguous forest sector.

Pct1OPch is percent of hexagon in one nonforest sector.

A listing of this dataset from a space-delimited text (.txt) file as would be appropriate for input to **R** appears in Appendix 1.

Architecture of R

As mentioned in our opening paragraph, Appendices 2–5 contain tutorials on **R**. We also note at the outset that a working folder for files should be set up on the computer and data files transferred to it before starting **R**. The **R** menu bar allows for changing to that working directory at the beginning of an **R** session so that all data files will be directly accessible. Any previous work in **R** can likewise be reloaded if it was saved in concluding a prior session. Versions of **R** from 2.7.2 and later have been used here. The file name used here for the data described above is BAMBI.txt which reflects its content of Bird And Mammal Biodiversity Information. Direct preparation of such data files should be done in a simple text editor like Microsoft Notepad instead of a more sophisticated word processor that would corrupt the file by inclusion of formatting information. A special component of **R** documentation provides guidance for Import/Export from and to other software environments, such as spreadsheets (R Data Import/Export, 2005, R Development Core Team, ISBN 3-900051-10-0).

The first task is to get data into R so that analysis can be initiated. When working with a tabular matrix of data as variate values for cases, the **R** construct of a *data frame* is most useful. A *data frame* is one among several kinds of analytical *objects* upon which **R** can operate. The user gives names to objects in **R**, and the objects are effectively addressed by name as far as the user is concerned (Dalgaard 2002; Allerhand 2011; Curran 2011). Appendix 6 is a glossary of the more important names used for present purposes. **R** (mostly) does not use capital (upper case) letters in its preset syntax, so the user can help to avoid conflict with existing things in the language by having one or more capital letters in each name. However, there are some very notable exceptions, particularly T as TRUE and F as FALSE. TRUE and FALSE should never be reassigned. If T and F are used otherwise for notational consistency, they must be reset before use in command function calls.

R works with expressions entered in response to prompts. The default prompt is a> "greater than" sign, which is also used frequently otherwise in the **R** syntax. If a command is incomplete at the end of a line, **R** issues a continuation prompt for which the default is a+ "plus" sign that is likewise used frequently otherwise. The option is also provided to change these prompts, and the convention here will be to use a single @ as the main prompt and a double @@ as the continuation prompt. This is accomplished with the **R** command—

```
options(prompt="@ ",continue="@@ ")
```

Following is an initial **R** session to transfer data from the BAMBI.txt file as a data frame named BAMBI, then to list first the names of variates in the file, then the last six cases.

```
@ # Get data as a data frame named BAMBI.
@ # Note use of T in the following function call.
@ BAMBI <- read.table("BAMBI.txt",header=T)
@ names(BAMBI)
[1] "HexNo"   "BirdSp" "MamlSp" "ElevSD" "PctFor" "PctlFPch" "PctlOPch"
@ tail(BAMBI)
    HexNo BirdSp MamlSp ElevSD PctFor PctlFPch PctlOPch
206  4310    120     43     37   37.5     22.3     31.8
207  4311    109     43     31   23.9      8.7     73.0
208  4312     63     41     27   17.6     17.6     76.1
209  4442    105     41     33   42.6     34.2     27.5
210  4443    126     43     42   54.0     32.8     36.6
211  4444    113     43     16   66.5     57.9     26.2
```

Note first that commentary can be incorporated in an **R** session by starting it with a "hash mark" # symbol. Everything on the line following # will be ignored by **R**. Also note that the specifications for an **R** command are placed in parentheses following the command "word" and separated by commas. The two-character symbol < - is conveniently thought of as "put into". In this situation, it puts the result of the read.table command into a data frame object named BAMBI.

Command words will not contain spaces, but can have periods as connectors to convey a multiword sense of meaning as in the read.table command. Command specifications in parentheses are interpreted by default order or by keyword. For this read.table command, the default is to put the file name as the first specification. The header = T is used to declare that it is true that column names are present in the first line of the file as header information prior to the actual data lines. There is a default condition for some specifications that can be omitted when the default pertains. Note particularly that the hexagon identification numbers are being allowed to have a place in the data frame in the manner of a variate. This will require that the column be explicitly excluded from computations in which it does not belong. It would also have been possible to add a specification that the first item for each case be used as a row name instead of a variate, with the added specification being –

```
BAMBI<- read.table("BAMBI.txt",header=T,row.names=1)
```

The hexagon identifiers would then be treated as names rather than numbers, and there would not be sequential numbers for cases appearing in output from the tail() command. Listing the last half-dozen cases in the file allows one to verify that there are the expected number of cases and that they have been read properly. If desired, the first half-dozen cases could have been similarly listed with the head() command.

In order to avoid the necessity of excluding the column of hexagon IDs for each calculation, the first thing will be to make a subsidiary data frame named BAMBIV that contains only the variates. This is accomplished by specifying that the first column containing IDs be eliminated in transferring information from the BAMBI data frame to the BAMBIV data frame. Excluding a component of a data frame requires knowing how **R** designates different components of a data frame. This is done in terms of rows and columns placed in square brackets with rows first and columns second using a comma to separate rows from columns. Anything not specified is taken as being included. A single row or column can be excluded by specifying its number as negative. The command

```
BAMBIV<- BAMBI[,-1]
```

thus serves to create the reduced data frame. It is also prudent to use the length() command to verify that numbers of rows and columns in the data frame are as expected.

```
@ BAMBI<- read.table("BAMBI.txt",header=T)
@ BAMBIV<- BAMBI[,-1]
@ length(BAMBIV)
[1] 6
@ length(BAMBIV[,1])
[1] 211
```

It can be seen that the default for the length() command is to give the number of columns in a data frame, but asking for the length of a particular column will give the number of rows (cases) in the data frame.

Throughout the ensuing presentation, heavy reliance will be placed on the help facilities of **R** for making the mathematical specifics of computational commands available to the reader. An **R** command with its defaults is effectively a complete mathematical specification, and including optional arguments will alter the analytical scenario in specific ways. It is always advisable for users to avail themselves of the help facilities to ensure that their understanding of what a command will do is correct. Giving extensive mathematical formulas here would be redundant, since we exercise and interpret the results of each command we use. It should become obvious in what follows that many **R** commands are composite codes for sophisticated analytical scenarios.

The help facilities of **R** are simple to invoke, but the help itself is sometimes terse. If a command is known, help on that command can be obtained by prefixing a question mark. Thus, ?help gives help on the help command, with help(help) being an equivalent form. The help itself will appear in a pop-up hypertext window on the **R** desktop. The standard help facilities include brief examples of the command, but there is some circularity in that one must know the command in order to obtain help on it. This can sometimes be circumvented by having **R** search its help texts for words that pertain to a desired command. The form for this is:

```
help.search("target text")
```

and in response, **R** will indicate which commands use those words in their explanatory help text.

R sometimes extends the meaning of mathematical terms. For example, a *vector* object in **R** is any singly ordered set of the same kind of quantities. One might, therefore, expect that multiplying two vector objects would give their inner product.

```
@ Twos <- rep(2,5)
@ Threes <- rep(3,5)
@ TwosTimesThrees <- Twos * Threes
@ TwosTimesThrees
[1] 6 6 6 6 6
@ TwosTimesThrees <- Twos %*% Threes
@ TwosTimesThrees
     [,1]
[1,]   30
```

However, the snippet of **R** code does not conform to that expectation. Twos is a vector object created by repeating the number 2 five times, and Threes is a vector object created by repeating the number 3 five times. Use of the conventional asterisk symbol * as a multiplication operator causes the computation of element-by-element products. A special multiplication operator %*% gives the inner (vector) product. Notice also that **R** did not distinguish whether or not one vector was a row vector and the other a column vector. **R** presents the result as a matrix object having one row and one column.

References

Allerhand M (2011) A tiny handbook of R. Springer, New York

Balakrishnan N, Ng HKT (2009) Precedence-type tests for the comparison of treatments with a control. In: Glaz J, Pozdnyakov V, Wallenstein S (eds) Scan statistics: methods and applications. Birkhauser, Boston, MA, pp 27–54

Brüggemann R, Patil GP (2011) Ranking and prioritization for multi-indicator systems. Springer, New York

Crawley M (2007) The R book. Wiley, Chichester

Curran J (2011) Introduction to data analysis with R for forensic scientists. Taylor & Francis/CRC, Boca Raton, FL

Dalgaard P (2002) Introductory statistics with R. Springer, New York

Hogan T (2010) Bare-bones R: a brief introductory guide. Sage, Los Angeles, CA

Horton N, Kleinman K (2011) Using R for data management, statistical analysis, and graphics. Taylor & Francis/CRC, Boca Raton, FL

Myers W, Bishop J, Brooks R, O'Connell T, Argent D, Storm G, Stauffer J Jr (2000) The Pennsylvania GAP analysis final report. The Pennsylvania State University, University Park, PA

R Development Core Team (2008) R: A language and environment for statistical computing. R Foundation for Statistical Computing, Vienna, Austria. ISBN 3-900051-07-0, URL http:// www.R-project.org/

Venables WN, Smith DM, the R Development Core Team (2005) An introduction to R. Network Theory Ltd, Bristol

Verzani J (2005) Using R for introductory statistics. Chapman & Hall/CRC, Boca Raton, FL

Part I
Synergistic Scalings, Contingent
Clustering and Distance Domains

Chapter 2
Suites of Scalings

The scales of measure for quantifying features of cases used in original recording of the data must obviously have some interpretive appeal; otherwise, they would not be used for recording the data in the beginning. In any case, the data as recorded on the original scales provide the starting point for rescaling to gain some comparative interpretive advantage. We pursue a structural scaling sequence of successive statistical simplification. In so doing, we focus on variability because variability consists of information and noise with (white) noise being variability that is lacking in pattern (independently random). A fairly crude gauge of variability is *range* as difference between maximum and minimum. Maximum and minimum are given in the default summary of a data frame provided by **R**.

```
@ summary(BAMBIV)
     BirdSp          MamlSp           ElevSD           PctFor
Min.   : 55.0   Min.   :34.00   Min.   : 11.00   Min.   :  8.60
1st Qu.:116.0   1st Qu.:42.00   1st Qu.: 40.00   1st Qu.: 53.65
Median :126.0   Median :46.00   Median : 68.00   Median : 74.20
Mean   :122.1   Mean   :45.16   Mean   : 72.45   Mean   : 69.95
3rd Qu.:131.0   3rd Qu.:48.00   3rd Qu.: 98.00   3rd Qu.: 89.25
Max.   :145.0   Max.   :53.00   Max.   :205.00   Max.   :100.00
    Pct1FPch         Pct1OPch
Min.   :  2.20   Min.   : 0.00
1st Qu.: 44.85   1st Qu.: 3.70
Median : 69.50   Median : 9.40
Mean   : 63.45   Mean   :18.30
3rd Qu.: 88.25   3rd Qu.:27.35
Max.   :100.00   Max.   :85.50
```

The quarter-point values (quartiles) of ordered cases also appear in the summary, with the *median* being the second quarter-point thus marking the middle as half of ordered values. The one remaining item that appears is the *mean* as the arithmetic average computed as total over all cases divided by the number of cases. **R** does not

W.L. Myers and G.P. Patil, *Multivariate Methods of Representing Relations in R for Prioritization Purposes*, Environmental and Ecological Statistics 6, DOI 10.1007/978-1-4614-3122-0_2, © Springer Science+Business Media, LLC 2012

subtract the minimum from the maximum for us. **R** commands are usually brief, but doing this series of simple subtractions does get a bit involved. We first get the means as a template for ranges, and then step through the variates incrementally in a "loop" procedure to get differences.

```
@ P <- length(BAMBIV)
@ BAMBIVmean <- mean(BAMBIV)
@ Ranges <- BAMBIVmean
@ for(I in 1:P) Ranges[I] <- max(BAMBIV[,I]) - min(BAMBIV[,I])
@ Ranges
  BirdSp   MamlSp   ElevSD   PctFor PctlFPch PctlOPch
    90.0     19.0    194.0     91.4     97.8     85.5
```

The first of these preceding lines puts the number of variates into an object named P. The second computes means for the variates. The third uses means as a template for ranges. The fourth uses an object named I as an incremental index to step through the variates putting the difference between the max and min values into the respective element of Ranges. Giving just the name of the Ranges object then displays its contents.

If we were to consider some sort of collective among these six variates, four of them would speak with similar voices since their differences between max and min are about 90. One would speak with a weak voice since it has only about ¼ of this range. The other would speak with an extra strong voice since its range is more than twice 90.

The disparities of variability are at least in part due to the different units of measure, which suggests that an alternative scaling might improve comparability. Before proceeding with alternative scalings, however, we are reminded that range is a somewhat simplistic expression of variability since it looks only at the most extreme values at the low and high ends. Further insight can be gained by looking also at sub-ranges, such as the range that encompasses the middle half of the values for the cases, called the *inter-quartile range* or **IQR** for short. It also helps to have a graphic comparison (Keen 2010), which can be obtained in the form of a **boxplot**. A boxplot is built around a box showing the ends of the inter-quartile range, and with a heavy line in the box at the median value that splits the cases into lower and upper halves. "Whiskers" extend above and below the box for a distance that is some multiple of the **IQR**, with the default being 1.5 times the **IQR**. Any cases having values beyond these whiskers are marked individually as what might be called "outliers". Boxplots for the BAMBIV variates are obtained as follows and shown in Fig. 2.1.

```
@ boxplot(BAMBIV)
```

The boxplots of Fig. 2.1 are quite revealing of differences in patterns of variability among the variates (Baclawski 2008; Oja 2010). The pattern of variability for mammal species is unique among these variates. Not only is the overall range small, but the range for the middle half of cases (**IQR**) is also small and there are no outliers. The basic message here is that many mammal species in the region are quite

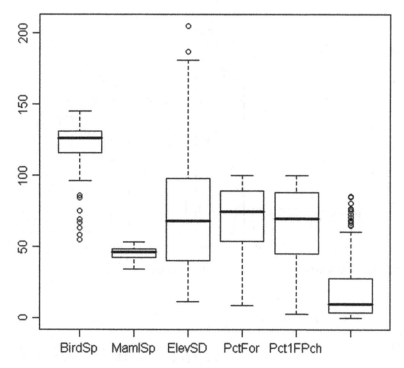

Fig. 2.1 Boxplots for variates in BAMBIV data frame

adaptable and accommodate heterogeneity of habitat. The other five variates have in common a skew character whereby there is a substantially heavier tail on one end or the other. The percent forest and percent in largest forest patch have quite similar patterns of variability with a heavier tail on the low side and no outliers. The elevation complexity has large overall variation, heavy tail on the high side, and a couple outliers on the high end. The other two variates have strong imbalance (skew) about the median line in the box along with several outliers, but the propensities are opposite for the two with the bird species being heavy on the low side and the percent of area in largest open patch being heavy on the high side.

Whereas the range responds only to changes in extremes, informational efficiency would entail change in response to alteration in any of the case values. This level of sensitivity is available in the *standard deviation* as an expression of variability, although not without sacrificing simplicity. The standard deviation is based on the average squared difference from the mean per degree of freedom, which is termed *variance*. In the straightforward situation of characterizing a random sample, the degrees of freedom are one less than the number of cases. The standard deviation is the square root of the variance and has the interpretive advantage of being expressed in the same units of measure as the case values, whereas variance is expressed in squared units of measure. Standard deviations are determined as follows and compared as a barplot in Fig. 2.2.

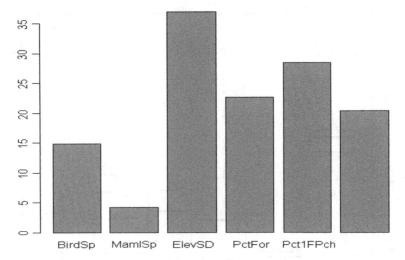

Fig. 2.2 Barplot of standard deviations for BAMBIV variates

```
@ BAMBIVsd <- sd(BAMBIV)
@ BAMBIVsd
    BirdSp     MamlSp     ElevSD     PctFor    Pct1FPch   Pct1OPch
 14.849153   4.165917  36.921159  22.588160  28.432770  20.311859
@ barplot(BAMBIVsd)
```

The standard deviation view in Fig. 2.2 is generally consistent with the features of the boxplot view from Fig. 2.1, but this single-value view of variability does not convey information about skewness or outliers. Thus, the boxplots are valuable despite the insensitivity of range as an expression of variability.

There is also another perspective on variability that can be considered, which is variability relative to average size. This is called *coefficient of variation* (**CV**) and expresses standard deviation as a percentage of the mean. A process for determining **CV** is much like that for determining range done earlier. This is accomplished as follows and displayed as a barplot in Fig. 2.3.

```
@ P <-length(BAMBIV)
@ BAMBIVsd <- sd(BAMBIV)
@ BAMBIVmean <- mean(BAMBIV)
@ BAMBIVcv <- BAMBIVsd
@ for(I in 1:P) BAMBIVcv[I] <-
@@ (BAMBIVsd[I]/BAMBIVmean[I]) * 100.0
@ BAMBIVcv
    BirdSp     MamlSp      ElevSD      PctFor    Pct1FPch    Pct1OPch
 12.156797   9.224561   50.964050   32.293725   44.809125  110.993765
@ barplot(BAMBIVcv)
```

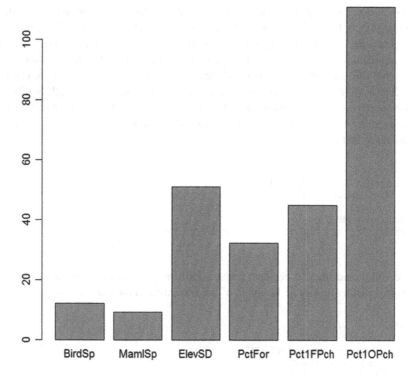

Fig. 2.3 Barplot of coefficient of variation for BAMBIV variates

It is apparent from comparing Figs. 2.2 and 2.3 that the pattern of variability relative to size of mean is quite different. The variability of bird species and mammal species is now quite similar, and the variability of elevation complexity is no longer notably large. The relative variability in percent of largest nonforest patch is about double that of any other variate.

Standardized Scaling as Universal Units

Thus, far we have examined different ways of gauging variability, but have not actually done any rescaling. We now consider **additive** and **multiplicative** rescaling, with particular attention to a commonly used version called *standardization*. By **additive rescaling**, we mean the addition (or subtraction) of the same constant value for all cases of a variate. By **multiplicative rescaling** we mean the multiplication (or division) of all cases for a variate by the same (nonzero) constant. We note, and it is easily proved, that additive rescaling will alter the mean for a variate by addition (or subtraction) of the additive value; but it does not alter the standard deviation. We also note that multiplicative rescaling will multiply both mean and standard deviation by the constant (Everitt and Hothorn 2006).

Standardized scaling expresses each variate in standard deviation units from the (original) mean. It consists of first subtracting the respective means, which changes all means to zero; then dividing by the respective standard deviations, which results in a standard deviation of 1.0 for all variates. Since the standard deviation used as a divisor has the same units (meters or whatever) as the original variates, there is unit cancellation so that the standardized data are dimensionless. From a slightly different perspective, standardization simplifies the scales for cross-comparison by universalizing the units of measure. Standardization can be accomplished with a single command as follows.

```
@ BAMBIVS <- scale(BAMBIV)
@ round(mean(BAMBIVS),digits=6)
  BirdSp   MamlSp   ElevSD   PctFor  Pct1FPch Pct10Pch
       0        0        0        0         0        0
@ round(sd(BAMBIVS),digits=6)
  BirdSp   MamlSp   ElevSD   PctFor  Pct1FPch Pct10Pch
       1        1        1        1         1        1
```

We will, however, also perform the standardization more mechanistically in the following manner and show boxplots of the standardized data in Fig. 2.4.

```
@ BAMBIV <- BAMBI[,-1]
@ P <- length(BAMBIV)
@ BAMBIVmean <- mean(BAMBIV)
@ BAMBIVsd <- sd(BAMBIV)
@ BAMBIS <- BAMBIV
@ for(I in 1:P) BAMBIS[,I] <- BAMBIV[,I] - BAMBIVmean[I]
@ for(I in 1:P) BAMBIS[,I] <- BAMBIS[,I]/BAMBIVsd[I]
@ BAMBISmean <- mean(BAMBIS)
@ BAMBISsd <- sd(BAMBIS)
@ round(BAMBISmean, 6)
  BirdSp   MamlSp   ElevSD   PctFor  Pct1FPch Pct10Pch
       0        0        0        0         0        0
@ round(BAMBISsd,6)
  BirdSp   MamlSp   ElevSD   PctFor  Pct1FPch Pct10Pch
       1        1        1        1         1        1
@ boxplot(BAMBIS)
```

The BAMBIS data frame for standardized data uses the BAMBIV data frame as a template. **R** effectively treats each column of a data frame as a vector, and the **R** protocol for subtracting a constant from a vector is to subtract the constant from each element, and likewise for dividing by a constant. Thus, the first "loop" subtracts the means and the second divides by the standard deviations. Since there is likely to be some small rounding error in **R** computations, the round() command is used to round the results to six places after the decimal for purposes of display.

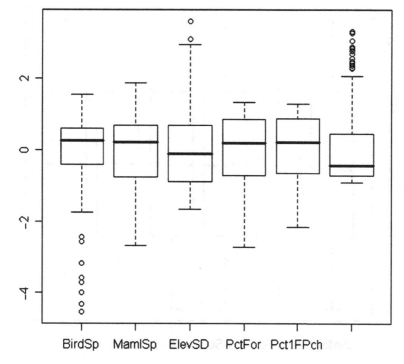

Fig. 2.4 Boxplot of standardized BAMBIS variates

Note, however, that rounding for display does not round the actual values in the vector being displayed. Boxplots in Fig. 2.4 show that the standardization does not remove the heavy-tailed characteristics or the outliers.

If the standardized data were to be multiplied through by some constant, this would change the standard deviation to the constant but nevertheless maintain the equality of variation. Likewise, adding some constant throughout would shift the means but leave the variation unchanged. Note also that coefficient of variation is undefined for standardized data because division by zero is not permitted. It also bears reemphasizing that standardization does not remove other distributional peculiarities, such as heavy-tailed skewness and outliers. In the ensuing presentation, such other distributional characteristics are considered as being structural features that may be of interest for understanding and interpreting the data.

Relative Rank Rescaling

A further structural simplification is to retain only the ordering information for cases by ranking. Apart from the effect of ties, this method of rescaling will equalize all other structural aspects of the distribution. Rank numbers assigned by **R** have the

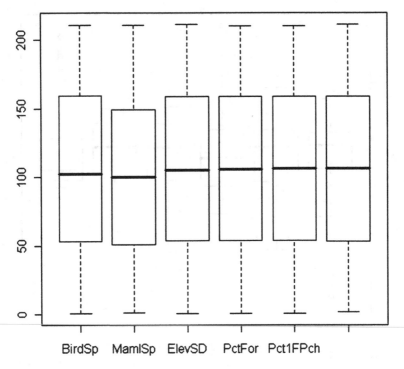

Fig. 2.5 Boxplot of ranks for BAMBIR variates

same sense as the original variates, with worst first. The following commands provide rank conversions of the BAMBI variates and boxplots in Fig. 2.5. The only evident difference among the ranked variates is that variability of mammal species has been slightly reduced by ties.

```
@ BAMBI <- read.table("BAMBI.txt",header=T)
@ BAMBIV <- BAMBI[,-1]
@ P <- length(BAMBIV)
@ BAMBIR <- BAMBIV
@ for(I in 1:P) BAMBIR[,I] <- rank(BAMBIV[,I],ties.method="average")
@ boxplot(BAMBIR)
@ mean(BAMBIR)
  BirdSp   MamlSp   ElevSD   PctFor Pct1FPch Pct1OPch
     106      106      106      106      106      106
@ sd(BAMBIR)
  BirdSp   MamlSp   ElevSD   PctFor Pct1FPch Pct1OPch
61.01067 60.79454 61.04854 61.05384 61.05388 61.05238
```

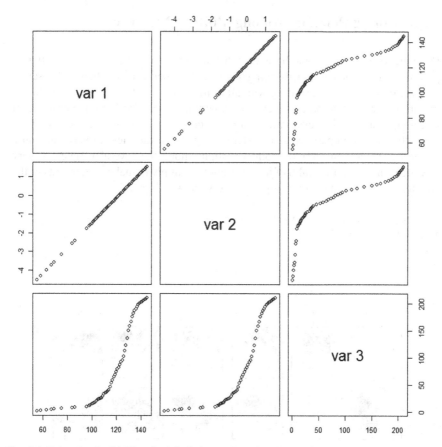

Fig. 2.6 Pairs plot for BirdSp of original observations (var 1), standardized scaling (var 2), and relative (regular) ranks (var3)

Note that ranks are the same whether they are determined from original observations or standardized data. A contrary sense of order comes from place ranks as opposed to regular ranks. First place is number 1 and best in place ranks, second place is number 2 and next best, and so on until the worst is reached at the highest rank number. Place ranks will be used later for prioritization purposes.

It is of interest at this juncture to use the cbind() capability of **R** for coupling columns along with the pairs() plotting procedure of lattice graphics to obtain a "checkerboard" of scatter plots for these three scalings. This is accomplished for BirdSp as follows and shown in Fig. 2.6.

```
@ pairs(cbind(BAMBIV[,1],BAMBIS[,1],BAMBIR[,1]))
```

The information retention by standardized scaling is evident in the straightline plot from corner to corner. Plots involving rank numbers on the vertical axis are seen to be essentially cumulative frequency distributions having the same shape for both original observations and standardized scaling.

Representing Relations Among Multiple Measures

From the foregoing, it should be evident that different ways of scaling serve different purposes rather one necessarily being analytically superior to another. In this sense, they are complementary, starting with all of the available structure of variability in the original observations and focusing on certain aspects with particular kinds of rescaling. Thus far, however, attention has been directed toward variates individually, albeit in a comparative sense. Here, we broaden the view to variability in a larger sense that considers the joint variation among the several variates. A very empirical entry into the realm of joint variation is simply to make scatter plots of the variates by pairs as shown for original observations in Fig. 2.7.

```
@ BAMBI <- read.table("BAMBI.txt",header=T)
@ BAMBIV <- BAMBI[,-1]
@ pairs(BAMBIV)
```

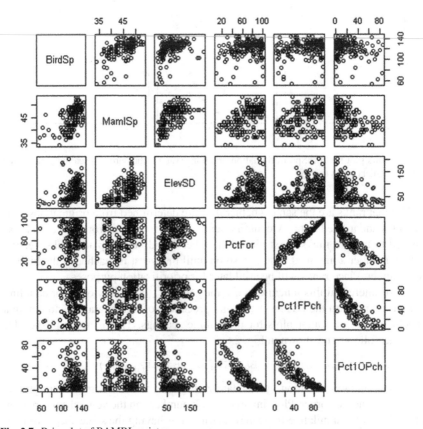

Fig. 2.7 Pairs plot of BAMBI variates

The idea of total variability among several variates becomes pertinent at this juncture. For several reasons that are not of immediate interest here, total variability is best approached in terms of squared standard deviations which are *variances* as noted earlier. In this sense, the sum of the squared standard deviations for a set of variates can be considered as *total variance* for the dataset. As shown below, this is 3332.243 for the BAMBIV variates. For standardized variates, total variance is always just the number of variates since the standard deviation and variance are both 1.0 for standardized data. If the units of measure are not the same for different variates, then one must always ask the question of how summation of variability in different units is to be interpreted. This question does not arise with standardized variates.

```
@ BAMBIVsd <- sd(BAMBIV)
@ TotalVar <- sum(BAMBIVsd^2)
@ TotalVar
[1] 3332.243
```

Another question arises as to what part of the total variance is due to joint variation among the variates, being in some sense redundant or multiple counting of the same underlying source of variation. As shown in Fig. 2.7, some of the variates are strongly related, such as percent forest and percent in one contiguous zone of forest, whereas relations are not obvious for some other pairs of variates. With this in mind, we proceed to work our way from variance to concepts of *covariance* and *correlation*.

We first calculate the numerator of a variance by two different but equivalent formulations using the percent forest variate as an example. The first formulation is the definitional one of sum of squared deviations from mean. The second uses sum of squared values and square of sum with only one subtraction. Both ways are then divided by degrees of freedom for variance (one less than number of cases) and the square root is taken to obtain the standard deviation that has already been calculated.

```
@ Numer8r1 <- sum((BAMBIV[,4]-mean(BAMBIV[,4]))^2)
@ Numer8r1
[1] 107147.2
@ Ncase <- length(BAMBIV[,4])
@ Numer8r2 <- sum(BAMBIV[,4]^2) - (sum(BAMBIV[,4])^2)/Ncase
@ Numer8r2
[1] 107147.2
@ Var1 <- Numer8r1 / (Ncase-1)
@ Var1
[1] 510.225
@ SD1 <- sqrt(Var1)
@ SD1
[1] 22.58816
@ Var2 <- Numer8r2 / (Ncase-1)
@ Var2
[1] 510.225
```

The foregoing results can also be compared directly with the result of using the built-in `var()` command.

```
@ var(BAMBIV[,4])
[1] 510.225
```

Since squaring a difference in the numerator of the variance provides an expression of variability for that variate, a parallel expression for joint variability of two variates is obtained by replacing the square with a product. The result of such replacement is called *covariance*. BAMBIV variates 4 and 5 (percent forest and forest patch) are illustrative, with results being compared to the built-in `cov()` command.

```
@ Numer8rA <-
@@ sum((BAMBIV[,4]-mean(BAMBIV[,4])) * (BAMBIV[,5]-mean(BAMBIV[,5])))
@ Numer8rA
[1] 130944.7
@ Numer8rB <-
@@ sum(BAMBIV[,4]*BAMBIV[,5]) - (sum(BAMBIV[,4])*sum(BAMBIV[,5]))/Ncase
@ Numer8rB
[1] 130944.7
@ CovA <- Numer8rA / (Ncase-1)
@ CovA
[1] 623.5462
@ CovB <- Numer8rB / (Ncase-1)
@ CovB
[1] 623.5462
@ cov(BAMBIV[,4],BAMBIV[,5])
[1] 623.5462
```

Applying the `cov()` command directly to a data frame gives a *covariance matrix* in which the value at the intersection of a particular row and column is the covariance for the respective variates, and the value at the intersection of like numbered rows and columns is the variance for that variate. A positive covariance indicates that the variates increase together (upward sloping trend line for a scatterplot); whereas a negative covariance indicates that one variate decreases as the other increases (downward sloping trend line for a scatterplot).

```
@ cov(BAMBIV)
             BirdSp     MamlSp      ElevSD      PctFor     Pct1FPch    Pct1OPch
BirdSp    220.49736   35.80478   194.94376    70.84607    79.40788   -72.48667
MamlSp     35.80478   17.35486    91.02787    45.44589    52.86664   -38.22190
ElevSD    194.94376   91.02787  1363.17202   378.00657   444.36957  -301.89381
PctFor     70.84607   45.44589   378.00657   510.22497   623.54617  -409.20433
Pct1FPch   79.40788   52.86664   444.36957   623.54617   808.42241  -502.85167
Pct1OPch  -72.48667  -38.22190  -301.89381  -409.20433  -502.85167   412.57162
```

The slope of the trend line for plotting a y-variate on the vertical against an x-variate on the horizontal is obtained by dividing the covariance of the two variates by the variance of the x-variate. The intercept of the trend line is obtained by multiplying the slope times mean(x) and then subtracting from mean(y). A scatter

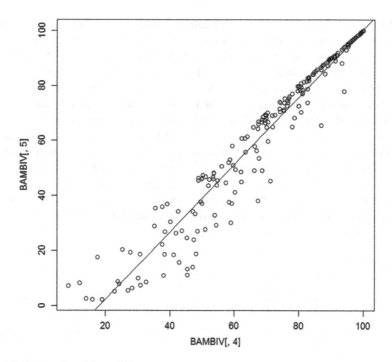

Fig. 2.8 Scatter plot with trend line

```
@ Slope4_5 <- cov(BAMBIV[,4],BAMBIV[,5]) / var(BAMBIV[,4])
@ Slope4_5
[1] 1.222100
@ Intercept4_5 <- mean(BAMBIV[,5]) - Slope4_5 * mean(BAMBIV[,4])
@ Intercept4_5
[1] -22.02792
@ plot(BAMBIV[,4],BAMBIV[,5])
@ abline(Intercept4_5,Slope4_5)
```

plot is obtained with the `plot()` command and a trend line with the `abline()` command as in Fig. 2.8.

The slope and intercept can also be obtained directly with the linear modeling `lm()` command (Fox 2002; Wright and London 2009).

```
@ lm(BAMBIV[,5] ~ BAMBIV[,4])

Call:
lm(formula = BAMBIV[, 5] ~ BAMBIV[, 4])

Coefficients:
(Intercept)   BAMBIV[, 4]
    -22.028         1.222
```

There is interpretive advantage in appealing to standardized variates for purposes of gauging relationship. This is because the covariance of standardized variates has a clearly delimited range of possibilities, which is between −1 and +1. A perfect positive relationship is indicated by +1, and −1 indicates a perfect inverse relationship. Zero indicates that no part of the variation is joint, so the variates have independent variation (no redundancy). These limits are intuitively clear by the fact that all standardized variates have both standard deviation and variance of 1.0 and a variate has perfect relationship (joint variation) with itself. Therefore, substituting another variate into the variance formulation to obtain covariance cannot yield a value having magnitude larger than the 1.0 value of the variance. Accordingly, the covariance of standardized variates has been given a special name as *correlation coefficient* and a built-in cor() command provided for calculation directly from the original data without having to do intermediate standardization. This is illustrated for the BAMBIS and BAMBIV variates as follows.

```
@ cov(BAMBIS)
              BirdSp      MamlSp      ElevSD      PctFor    Pct1FPch    Pct1OPch
BirdSp     1.0000000   0.5788003   0.3555759   0.2112191   0.1880800  -0.2403293
MamlSp     0.5788003   1.0000000   0.5918184   0.4829511   0.4463258  -0.4517020
ElevSD     0.3555759   0.5918184   1.0000000   0.4532556   0.4233015  -0.4025587
PctFor     0.2112191   0.4829511   0.4532556   1.0000000   0.9708868  -0.8918867
Pct1FPch   0.1880800   0.4463258   0.4233015   0.9708868   1.0000000  -0.8707050
Pct1OPch  -0.2403293  -0.4517020  -0.4025587  -0.8918867  -0.8707050   1.0000000
@ cor(BAMBIV)
              BirdSp      MamlSp      ElevSD      PctFor    Pct1FPch    Pct1OPch
BirdSp     1.0000000   0.5788003   0.3555759   0.2112191   0.1880800  -0.2403293
MamlSp     0.5788003   1.0000000   0.5918184   0.4829511   0.4463258  -0.4517020
ElevSD     0.3555759   0.5918184   1.0000000   0.4532556   0.4233015  -0.4025587
PctFor     0.2112191   0.4829511   0.4532556   1.0000000   0.9708868  -0.8918867
Pct1FPch   0.1880800   0.4463258   0.4233015   0.9708868   1.0000000  -0.8707050
Pct1OPch  -0.2403293  -0.4517020  -0.4025587  -0.8918867  -0.8707050   1.0000000
```

To calculate correlation from original data, one first calculates covariance and then divides by the product of the standard deviations, as illustrated for percent forest and forest patch (variates 4 and 5).

```
@ COVAR <- cov(BAMBIV[,4],BAMBIV[,5])
@ COVAR
[1] 623.5462
@ CORL8 <- COVAR / (sd(BAMBIV[,4]) * sd(BAMBIV[,5]))
@ CORL8
[1] 0.9708868
```

Slope of trend line is calculated by multiplying correlation by the standard deviation of the *y*-variate and dividing by the standard deviation of the *x*-variate, as follows for comparison with the result obtained earlier.

```
@ SLOPE <- CORL8 * ((sd(BAMBIV[,5])) / (sd(BAMBIV[,4])))
@ SLOPE
[1] 1.222100
```

Correlation as presented above is formally called the *Pearson correlation coefficient*. It is also possible to make use of rank scaling in a relational way by calculating correlation from ranked data instead of original data or standardized data. This latter is called the *Spearman rank correlation coefficient*. The Spearman correlation is unaffected by certain types of curvilinearity in the scatter plot relation, but it still must lie within the −1 to +1 range. The cor() command can also be modified with an optional argument to calculate Spearman rank correlations directly from the original data.

```
@ cor(BAMBIR)
              BirdSp       MamlSp      ElevSD       PctFor     Pct1FPch     Pct1OPch
BirdSp     1.0000000    0.5790877   0.4339592    0.1648744    0.1638723   -0.1164442
MamlSp     0.5790877    1.0000000   0.6298376    0.4926405    0.4640142   -0.4595067
ElevSD     0.4339592    0.6298376   1.0000000    0.4495578    0.4245905   -0.3896729
PctFor     0.1648744    0.4926405   0.4495578    1.0000000    0.9826981   -0.9344544
Pct1FPch   0.1638723    0.4640142   0.4245905    0.9826981    1.0000000   -0.9303386
Pct1OPch  -0.1164442   -0.4595067  -0.3896729   -0.9344544   -0.9303386    1.0000000

@ cor(BAMBIV,method="spearman")
              BirdSp       MamlSp      ElevSD       PctFor     Pct1FPch     Pct1OPch
BirdSp     1.0000000    0.5790877   0.4339592    0.1648744    0.1638723   -0.1164442
MamlSp     0.5790877    1.0000000   0.6298376    0.4926405    0.4640142   -0.4595067
ElevSD     0.4339592    0.6298376   1.0000000    0.4495578    0.4245905   -0.3896729
PctFor     0.1648744    0.4926405   0.4495578    1.0000000    0.9826981   -0.9344544
Pct1FPch   0.1638723    0.4640142   0.4245905    0.9826981    1.0000000   -0.9303386
Pct1OPch  -0.1164442   -0.4595067  -0.3896729   -0.9344544   -0.9303386    1.0000000
```

An interesting but unconventional way of visualization when exploring the correlations of a particular variate with the others is to make a barplot of the corresponding column in the correlation matrix. For example, the correlations of BirdSp with the other variates are shown in Fig. 2.9 as obtained from the command:

```
@ barplot(cor(BAMBIS)[,1])
```

It is seen from Fig. 2.9 that the two most substantial relations for BirdSp are first with MamlSp and to a lesser degree with ElevSD. The inclusion of a bar for BirdSp is not without purpose since it gives a bar of perfect correlation for visual comparison. The corresponding view for MamlSp is shown in Fig. 2.10 where relations are seen with most of the variates. The inverse influence of large open areas becomes evident for both birds and mammals.

A similar strategy can be used to show the difference in strength between Spearman correlation and Pearson correlation, shown for MamlSp in Fig. 2.11 as obtained from the command:

```
@ barplot((cor(BAMBIR)-cor(BAMBIS))[,2],ylim=c(-1,1))
```

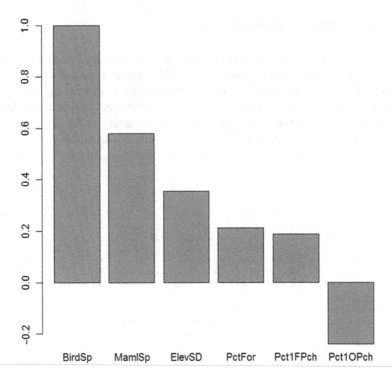

Fig. 2.9 Barplot of correlations for BirdSp with other variates

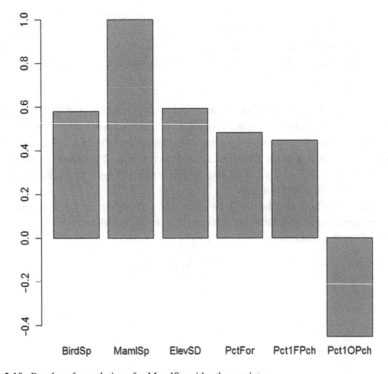

Fig. 2.10 Barplot of correlations for MamlSp with other variates

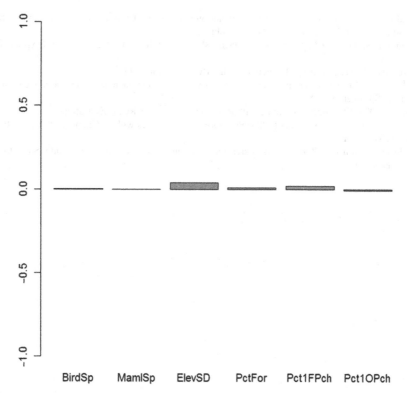

Fig. 2.11 Barplot of nonlinear relational effects on correlation for MamlSp

where there is little evidence of nonlinear relational effects. Note that it is necessary to control the vertical scale in this situation, with `c(-1,1)` serving to concatenate the desired lower and upper limits.

Additional references that may be helpful for utilizing **R** in such statistical settings are Crawley (2005); Maindonald and Braun (2007); Murrell (2006); Rizzo (2008); Ugarte et al. (2008); and Marques de Sa (2007).

References

Baclawski K (2008) Introduction to probability with R. Chapman & Hall/CRC, Boca Raton, FL
Crawley M (2005) Statistics: an introduction using R. Wiley, Chichester
Everitt B, Hothorn T (2006) A handbook of statistical analysis using R. Chapman & Hall/CRC, Boca Raton, FL
Fox J (2002) An R and S-Plus companion to applied regression. Sage, Thousand Oaks, CA
Keen K (2010) Graphics for statistics and data analysis with R. Chapman & Hall/CRC, Boca Raton, FL

Maindonald J, Braun J (2007) Data analysis and graphics using R: an example-based approach, 2nd edn. Cambridge University Press, Cambridge

Marques de Sa J (2007) Applied statistics: using SPSS, STATISTICA, MATLAB and R. Springer, New York

Murrell P (2006) R graphics. Chapman & Hall/CRC, Boca Raton, FL

Oja H (2010) Multivariate nonparametric methods with R: an approach based on spatial signs and ranks. Springer, New York

Rizzo M (2008) Statistical computing with R. Chapman & Hall/CRC, Boca Raton, FL

Ugarte M, Militino A, Arnholt A (2008) Probability and statistics with R. Chapman & Hall/CRC, Boca Raton, FL

Wright D, London K (2009) Modern regression techniques using R: a practical guide. Sage, Los Angeles, CA

Chapter 3
Rotational Rescaling and Disposable Dimensions

The scalings done thus far have treated the variates individually and have been of a relatively simple nature, i.e., either additive, multiplicative, or ranking. We now proceed to considering the data jointly among variates as a constellation of points in multidimensional space having as many perpendicular axes as there are variates (Manly 1998; Krzanowski 2000; Anderson 2003). A point along an axis one unit from the origin provides a *basis case* or *basis vector* for that axis. This is effectively an "artificial" point having a coordinate of 1.0 on that axis and 0.0 on all other axes. An additive rescaling shifts the constellation of points upward or downward relative to the respective axis. A multiplicative rescaling changes the *magnitudes* of values on an axis, thus effectively stretching or compressing the axis and expanding or shrinking the constellation of points relative to that axis. It is also possible (and useful) to consider rigidly *rotating* the axial framework itself, which does not change the overall multidimensional shape of the constellation and does not change the (Euclidian) distances between points but does give a different perspective view as seen along an axis. The rotational rescaling consists of determining the value along a repositioned axis at which a perpendicular projection of each data point will impinge on the new axis.

Coordinates of data points (cases) on a rotated axis are determined as a composite of weighted components from the variates. The composite has the form:

$$c_1 x_{i1} + c_2 x_{i2} + \cdots + c_p x_{ip}$$

where in x_{ij} is the jth variate value for the ith case, and c_j is the weight coefficient. The c_j weight is the cosine of the angle that the new axis makes with the jth variate (unrotated) axis, and is thus called a *direction cosine*. A geometric requirement is that the squares of the direction cosines sum to one, and any set of weight coefficients that satisfy this requirement can be interpreted geometrically as defining a rotated axis. If a set of weight coefficients does not satisfy this requirement, it can be broken down into a rotation followed by a multiplicative change of magnitude.

To separate the rotation from the change of magnitude, first calculate the magnitude change factor as the square root of the sum of the squared coefficients and then find the direction cosines as weights by dividing each coefficient by the magnitude factor. As an example, using one-sixth as a coefficient for the BAMBI variates would provide an "averaging" axis. However, the sum of squares for these coefficients is also one-sixth, so they do not provide a simple rotation. The square root of one-sixth is 0.4082482 so this is the factor by which magnitude is reduced after rotation. Dividing one-sixth by this factor also gives 0.4082482 as the rotational weighting coefficients. Six times the square of 0.4082482 is 1.0 as required for simple rotation. Although easy enough to do mathematically, adding together components having different units does not give a result that is straightforward to interpret. Such interpretive issues do not arise if the variates have been standardized to render them in universal units (or without units).

Principal Component Composites

Composites of components as introduced in the previous section can be interpretively advantageous in several regards. It would simplify interpretive tasks if the variability inherent in a dataset could be recast into axial dimensions with each axis autonomous in the sense of not having any relation (correlation) to the other axial dimensions. By a multivariate optimization approach, it can be proven that there is a unique rigid rotation which accomplishes this. Since it is a rigid rotation of axes, it does not alter the multidimensional shape of the constellation of data points and thus preserves the total variability of the data and the (Euclidean) distances between data points. Although it may not be immediately obvious, this preservation implies that the sum of the variances for the rotated (composite) axes is equal to the sum of variances for the variates prior to rotation. Due to the optimality properties of this rotation, it is known as *principal component analysis* (PCA) and the resulting axial composite variates are called *principal components* or *principal axes* (McGarigal et al. 2000; Podani 2000). Despite the impression that is conveyed by some treatments of principal components, these optimality and independence properties do not depend upon the input variates conforming to any particular statistical distribution. However, it is true that probability statements arising from many tests of significance for the components depend rather heavily on the type of distribution.

It is perhaps an understatement to say that the principal component analytical process is not simple, and in Part III of this book we will be much more specific about that computational process. However, **R** makes it possible to obtain principal components in a one-line command (Everitt 2005). The most fundamental output of principal components analysis would be the set of weighting coefficients for combining input variates into composite components, with each set serving to produce one of the composite (principal) components. Most frequently, however, composite components are calculated internally and a dataset of principal component (score) values is provided as the rescaled result. A standardization of input data is often conducted as a preliminary phase of the principal component process. If standardized data are used directly as inputs, then this internal standardization phase will have no effect since standardized data will not be altered by standardization. Doing PCA on the standardized variates of the BAMBI data gives:

```
@ BAMBISpca <- princomp(BAMBIS,cor=T,scores=T)
@ BAMBISpca

Call:
princomp(x = BAMBIS, cor = T, scores = T)

Standard deviations:
   Comp.1     Comp.2     Comp.3     Comp.4     Comp.5     Comp.6
1.9034614  1.1324809  0.7745351  0.5674372  0.3814361  0.1641295

6 variables and 211 observations.

@ summary(BAMBISpca)

Importance of components:
                           Comp.1     Comp.2     Comp.3      Comp.4      Comp.5
Standard deviation     1.9034614  1.1324809  0.7745351  0.56743722  0.38143612
Proportion of Variance 0.6038609  0.2137521  0.0999841  0.05366417  0.02424892
Cumulative Proportion  0.6038609  0.8176131  0.9175972  0.97126133  0.99551025
                           Comp.6
Standard deviation     0.164129505
Proportion of Variance 0.004489749
Cumulative Proportion  1.000000000

@ attributes(BAMBISpca)
$names
[1] "sdev"      "loadings" "center"    "scale"     "n.obs"     "scores"
"call"
$class
[1] "princomp"

@ PCAvars <- BAMBISpca$sdev^2
@ PCAvars
     Comp.1     Comp.2      Comp.3      Comp.4      Comp.5      Comp.6
3.62316546  1.28251288  0.59990466  0.32198500  0.14549351  0.02693849
@ sum(PCAvars)
[1] 6
```

Specifying cor=T requests a preliminary standardization, and scores=T requests that the values for the data cases on the rotated axes be computed. The result is an **R** object of the class "princomp," which is a compound object.

A little information about the compound object is provided in response to the name of the object, giving the standard deviations of the principal component (score) rotated variates. By convention, the principal component variates are given in order of decreasing standard deviation throughout the compound object. A summary of the compound object provides additional information about the variability of the principal components, with the first line again being the standard deviations. The standard deviations are then squared and summed to obtain a total variance as a base for calculating proportions. The second line of the summary gives the fraction of the total variance that is attributable to each principal component, and the third line cumulates these from first to last principal component. Thus, it can be seen that the first five components account for 99.6% of the variability in the (standardized) data, and consequently most of the major messages that the data have to convey will reside in the first five principal components.

While the summary tells us something about the comparative nature of the principal components, it does not tell about the objects that comprise the compound object. This information can be obtained by the attributes() command, which tells us the names of the objects and the class of the compound object. The "sdev" object consists of the standard deviations that are given by the summary. The **R** approach to principal components uses the term "loadings" for the weight coefficients (direction cosines) of rotation, as explained earlier. The case values as coordinates on the rotated (principal component) axes are the "scores."

An object within a compound object is accessed by appending the object name to the compound name with a dollar sign. This protocol is illustrated above in squaring the standard deviations to obtain the variances, which are not given in the summary.

These variances are quite informative when PCA is done on standardized data, whereupon the variances sum to the number of variates. If all variates carried an equal "share" of the information on variability, they would all have a variance of one. Since principal components are unraveling the redundancies in the data, principal component variates having variance greater than one reflect aspects of the data that had some element of redundancy among the recorded variates. Variances equal to or somewhat less than one reflect separate aspects of information remaining after the removal of redundancies. Variances near zero reflect minor aspects of the data in which little remains after the removal of redundancies. Accordingly, it is clear that the first two principal components reflect aspects having some redundancy. The second two components reflect aspects having a modest amount of information after removing redundancies. It is questionable whether the fifth component embodies a substantial message, but it is worth examining further before possibly deciding that it is a disposable dimension. It often helps to have a graphic called a *scree plot* in making such assessments (Fig. 3.1).

```
@ screeplot(BAMBISpca,type="lines")
```

"Scree" is the name given to stony rubble that falls down and piles up at the base of a steep rocky slope. The shape of the scree plot is reminiscent of how the scree piles up deeper near the slope face and then thins going farther away.

It is always a good precautionary measure to examine the first few lines of a rescaled dataset with the head() command, and also to verify the anticipated aggregate proprieties. This applies to the principal component scores, and an aggregate anticipation is that the scores will be uncorrelated. The leading scores are as follows:

```
@ head(BAMBISpca$scores)
        Comp.1     Comp.2     Comp.3     Comp.4      Comp.5       Comp.6
[1,]   4.9955961 -3.143884 -1.7936443 -0.7239916 -0.67044694 -0.241477534
[2,]   1.3069029 -4.571346 -1.4029274 -0.6646216  0.12999705  0.000879196
[3,]   2.1753114 -0.962393  0.6321927  0.8459550  0.12009576 -0.178545602
[4,]   4.6242030 -1.088564 -0.3369930  0.5429365 -0.31479765 -0.230842574
[5,]  -0.1122134 -3.721707 -0.5501783  0.4252278 -0.20011708  0.126752824
[6,]   0.5869564 -1.446075  0.7873307  0.7133432 -0.06085062 -0.075098795
```

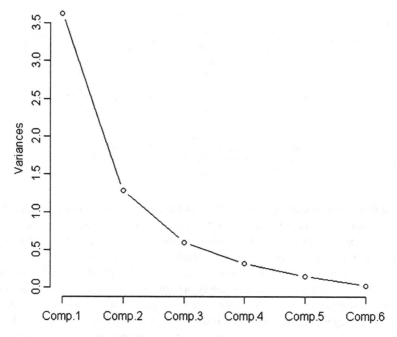

Fig. 3.1 Scree plot of decline in principal component variances for BAMBISpca

Verification of the uncorrelated condition to four places after the decimal is:

```
@ round(cor(BAMBISpca$scores),4)
        Comp.1 Comp.2 Comp.3 Comp.4 Comp.5 Comp.6
Comp.1     1      0      0      0      0      0
Comp.2     0      1      0      0      0      0
Comp.3     0      0      1      0      0      0
Comp.4     0      0      0      1      0      0
Comp.5     0      0      0      0      1      0
Comp.6     0      0      0      0      0      1
```

It is likewise informative to examine the loadings as weighting coefficients from which the principal component scores are computed. However, the default method for printing loadings is not ideal, so an explicit print command with specifications is used.

```
@ print(BAMBISpca$loadings,digits=6,cutoff=.0000001)
Loadings:
          Comp.1     Comp.2     Comp.3     Comp.4     Comp.5     Comp.6
BirdSp   -0.246991  0.631041  0.585503  0.437640 -0.080006  0.006253
MamlSp   -0.382424  0.450733 -0.041235 -0.804472  0.031298 -0.027142
ElevSD   -0.350360  0.325290 -0.785458  0.391019  0.036855 -0.015358
PctFor   -0.482839 -0.308717  0.065256  0.015301 -0.324542  0.749493
Pct1FPch -0.471703 -0.336403  0.079175  0.035320 -0.475783 -0.656082
Pct1OPch  0.462988  0.290414 -0.167375 -0.083178 -0.812136  0.082492

                 Comp.1    Comp.2    Comp.3    Comp.4    Comp.5    Comp.6
SS loadings    1.000000 1.000000 1.000000 1.000000 1.000000 1.000000
Proportion Var 0.166667 0.166667 0.166667 0.166667 0.166667 0.166667
Cumulative Var 0.166667 0.333333 0.500000 0.666667 0.833333 1.000000
```

The first part gives the weight coefficients for each component in a column. The first line of the second part shows that the sum of squared weight coefficients for each principal component is 1.0 which satisfies the requirement for direction cosines. The remaining two lines are essentially not informative.

There is another feature that is noteworthy and would not otherwise be obvious. The weight coefficients are predominantly negative on all but the second and sixth principal component axes. This shows that the principal component process is definite with regard to orientation of a rotated axis, but is indifferent as to which end of the axis is positive or negative. Principal component axes become more interpretively intuitive if all the signs are reversed for any axis which has predominantly negative loadings.

Orientation of principal components relative to parent variates can be seen from biplots, along with perspectives on relations among parent variates. One of two aspects of a biplot consists of a scatter plot of cases on two of the principal component axes. The second aspect of a biplot arises from rotating a basis case for each of the parent variates and plotting an arrow in that direction. The directional components for variates on principal component axes are simply the weight coefficients (loadings) in the column for the respective principal component axis. The magnitudes (lengths) of the arrows can be chosen for a good fit on the graph or used to convey some other aspect of variability. Arrows closer together (smaller angles) are more strongly correlated (Fig. 3.2).

```
@ biplot(BAMBISpca,choices=c(1,2),cex=c(0.6,0.8),col=c(1,1))
```

It can be seen from Fig. 3.2 that the arrows for all standardized variates except nonforest patch point toward the negative end of the scale for the first principal component. All of the (de)forestation variates are closely related with respect to the first two components since they lie almost along a straight line. The choices() specification of the biplot command determines which two components are to be plotted. The cex() specification controls the size of labels for points and arrows. The col() specification determines colors for plotting, with default being to plot the arrows in red. It is usually advisable to make biplots for pairings of at least the first three components (see Figs. 3.3 and 3.4).

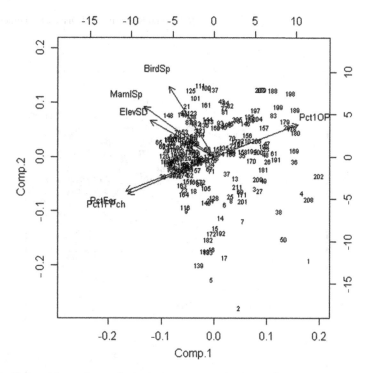

Fig. 3.2 Biplot of first and second principal components for BAMBIS variates

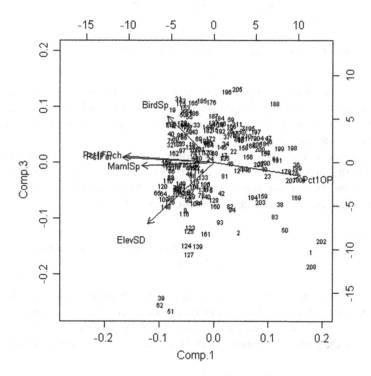

Fig. 3.3 Biplot of first and third principal components for BAMBIS variates

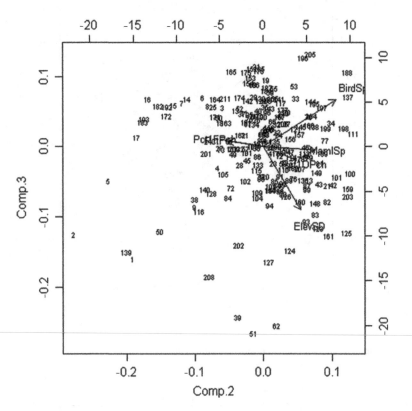

Fig. 3.4 Biplot of second and third principal components for BAMBIS variates

Perspective on relationship from a biplot can shift with choice of components to plot. The (de)forestation variates still appear closely related in Fig. 3.3, but the other three have shifted with mammal species also being close to the forest variates, whereas this was not the case in Fig. 3.2.

Case numbers in the biplots are quite convenient for identifying outliers, but get garbled in the more densely populated parts of the scatter plot. To obtain hexagon ID corresponding to a case number, we need only display the respective line of the BAMBI data frame. For the example of case number 51 this is:

```
@ BAMBI[51,]
   HexNo BirdSp MamlSp ElevSD PctFor PctlFPch PctlOPch
51  2524    103     48    187   94.1     77.8      2.1
```

With this introduction to principal component scaling, we are ready to make a data frame of the data scaled as principal component scores, change signs as appropriate, and investigate the structural characteristics of the data (Joe 1997) that are exhibited in the principal component (PC) axes. First, we make the data frame:

```
@ BAMBISpc <- BAMBISpca$scores
@ BAMBISpc <- as.data.frame(BAMBISpc)
```

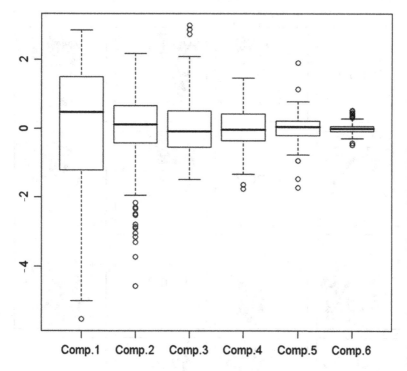

Fig. 3.5 Boxplots of BAMBISpc-modified principal component scaling

Next, we reverse the positive and negative ends of the axes (reverse the signs) for principal components 1, 3, and 5 for better correspondence to the parent (standardized) variates.

```
@ BAMBISpc[,1] <- -1.0 * BAMBISpc[,1]
@ BAMBISpc[,3] <- -1.0 * BAMBISpc[,3]
@ BAMBISpc[,5] <- -1.0 * BAMBISpc[,5]
```

We then begin to investigate the structural characteristics of the data as seen in principal components by making boxplots (Fig. 3.5) along with paired scatter plots for major principal components (Fig. 3.6) and for the minor components (Fig. 3.7).

```
@ boxplot(BAMBISpc)
@ pairs(BAMBISpc[,1:4])
@ pairs(BAMBISpc[,5:6])
```

We are looking for evidence of substructure in examining these graphics, for which we can use a multivariate normal distribution as a reference. An unstructured (here taken as multivariate normal) dataset would have symmetrical boxplots largely lacking outliers, and scatter plots would appear as horizontally or vertically oriented

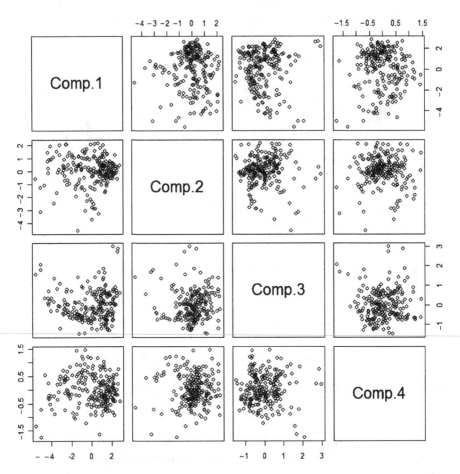

Fig. 3.6   Paired scatter plots for BAMBISpc principal components 1–4

ellipses with density of points grading off progressively from center symmetrically in both directions. This does not happen, so substructure is indicated.

One type of substructure is the presence of outliers, and the boxplots of Fig. 3.5 indicate the presence of outliers for several of the principal component variates. There is only one outlier for the (modified) first principal component, which is the minimum value as case number 202.

```
@ min(BAMBISpc)
[1] -5.526866
@ BAMBISpc[BAMBISpc$Comp.1<= -5.52686,]
        Comp.1       Comp.2     Comp.3       Comp.4     Comp.5       Comp.6
202 -5.526866 -0.5720659 1.576964 -1.334819 0.6708646 -0.4332491
```

For the second principal component, we need to find the lower whisker of the boxplot. Note that the IQR() command is one of the few exceptions that contain capital letters.

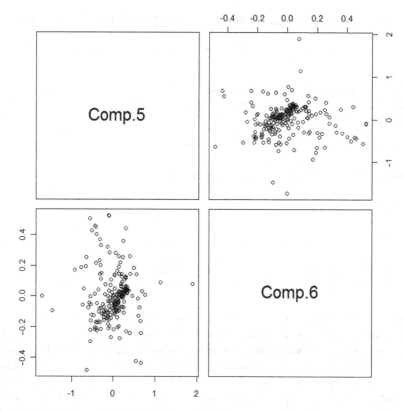

Fig. 3.7 Paired scatter plots for BAMBISpc principal components 5 and 6

```
@ quantile(BAMBISpc[,2],probs=0.25) - 1.5 * IQR(BAMBISpc[,2])
     25%
-2.056058
@ round(BAMBISpc[BAMBISpc$Comp.2<= -2.056,],4)
      Comp.1  Comp.2  Comp.3  Comp.4  Comp.5  Comp.6
1    -4.9956 -3.1439  1.7936 -0.7240  0.6704 -0.2415
2    -1.3069 -4.5713  1.4029 -0.6646 -0.1300  0.0009
5     0.1122 -3.7217  0.5502  0.4252  0.2001  0.1268
15   -0.0726 -2.1614 -0.6679  1.1609  0.0031  0.0060
16    0.1050 -2.7985 -0.7661  0.5727  0.2223  0.0944
17   -0.5411 -3.0517 -0.1520  0.4601  0.0396  0.1327
50   -3.6567 -2.4822  1.3513 -0.8873 -0.9336  0.1713
139   0.7821 -3.2957  1.6823 -1.6422  0.0289  0.0501
172   0.1345 -2.3301 -0.4883  0.5666  0.1933  0.0624
182   0.2781 -2.5161 -0.6539  0.5177  0.2690  0.1075
183   0.2856 -2.8976 -0.3984  0.3188  0.3054  0.1160
192  -0.3678 -2.3008 -0.6382  0.6462 -0.0144 -0.0122
193   0.4632 -2.8617 -0.4400  0.4212  0.2963  0.1271
```

For the third principal component, we need the upper whisker of the boxplot.

```
@ quantile(BAMBISpc[,3],probs=0.75) + 1.5 * IQR(BAMBISpc[,3])
     75%
2.098771
@ round(BAMBISpc[BAMBISpc$Comp.3>= 2.099,],4)
   Comp.1  Comp.2 Comp.3 Comp.4  Comp.5  Comp.6
39 2.6375 -0.5982 2.7246 0.2060  0.0768  0.0041
51 2.1579 -0.2293 2.9839 0.2017 -0.3002  0.3312
62 2.6901  0.3216 2.8672 0.7602 -0.0436 -0.0477
```

Outliers for the fourth principal component are:

```
@ quantile(BAMBISpc[,4],probs=0.25) - 1.5 * IQR(BAMBISpc[,4])
      25%
-1.530452
@ round(BAMBISpc[BAMBISpc$Comp.4<= -1.5305,],4)
     Comp.1  Comp.2 Comp.3  Comp.4 Comp.5  Comp.6
139  0.7821 -3.2957 1.6823 -1.6422 0.0289  0.0501
208 -5.0061 -1.2829 2.0843 -1.7542 0.5509 -0.4240
```

Interestingly, none of these sets of outliers on major axes have any cases in common. A second type of substructure consists of pronounced asymmetry, and again the boxplots give evidence of this. A third type of substructure involves noncentral regions of high density and/or notable locations of sparseness in the scatter plots, which are also evident from Figs. 3.6 and 3.7. Thus, the PCA suggests that there is one and possibly two disposable dimensions in this dataset and provides strong indications that major messages lie in the substructure. Clustering provides an analytical avenue for extracting these kinds of messages in the next chapter, with a primary goal being to discover what sets of data cases have distinctive characteristics (Podani 2000).

References

Anderson T (2003) An introduction to multivariate statistical analysis. Wiley-Interscience, New York
Everitt B (2005) An R and S-PLUS companion to multivariate analysis. Springer, London
Joe H (1997) Multivariate models and multivariate dependence concepts. Chapman & Hall/CRC, Boca Raton, FL
Krzanowski W (2000) Principles of multivariate analysis: a user's perspective. Oxford University Press, Oxford
Manly B (1998) Multivariate statistical methods: a primer. Chapman & Hall/CRC, Boca Raton, FL
McGarigal K, Cushman S, Stafford S (2000) Multivariate statistics for wildlife and ecology research. Springer, New York
Podani J (2000) Introduction to the exploration of multivariate biological data. Backhuys, Leiden

Chapter 4
Comparative Clustering for Contingent Collectives

Clustering creates collectives of cases that have similar properties with a degree of distinctiveness. Clustering requires some composite measure of similarity or disparity, a criterion for conformity among collectives (linkage), and a strategy for configuring collectives. The collectives produced by a clustering method are conventionally called *clusters*. There are many methods of clustering, however, which typically differ to some degree in the groupings that result (Abonyi and Balaz 2007; Everitt et al. 2001; Kaufman and Rousseeuw 1990; Xu and Wunsch 2009). It is by comparing the collectives produced by different methods of clustering that one can gain insight from inconsistencies and have some confidence relative to consistencies (Myers et al. 2006). We call this comparative or complementary clustering and we use the term *contingents* (groups from groupings) for collectives of cases that emerge from this compound approach using cross-tabulations. Preliminary prioritization can be done among contingents and then progress to comparisons within contingents so that the computational complexities of comprehensive comparisons can be controlled.

There are multiple metrics of disparity, such as the Manhattan distance metric that simply sums the magnitudes of differences between cases across all axes and the Euclidian distance metric that is based on the sum of squares of differences across axes (Hardle and Simar 2007). The Euclidian distance metric is adopted here because it corresponds to the multidimensional extension of usual straight-line distance, and it is also invariant under rigid rotation of axes so that computation in a full principal component space is identical to computation in the (standardized) measurement space. This enables straightforward assessment of effect on substructure (Long et al. 2010) caused by disposing of dimensions corresponding to low-order principal component axes.

There are likewise multiple methods of linkage, such as single linkage (disparity of cases having least disparity), complete linkage (disparity of cases having greatest disparity), and average linkage (average of disparities for all possible pairings of cases). The Ward approach to linkage is used here because of its emphasis on compactness of collectives in a sum of squared distances sense (Podani 2000).

W.L. Myers and G.P. Patil, *Multivariate Methods of Representing Relations in R for Prioritization Purposes*, Environmental and Ecological Statistics 6, DOI 10.1007/978-1-4614-3122-0_4, © Springer Science+Business Media, LLC 2012

With regard to strategies for configuring collectives, we exploit those that **R** makes most readily available. This includes hierarchical agglomeration and k-means condensation (Lumley 2010).

Disparities and Dendrograms

The first concern is to tabulate disparities among the cases using the `dist()` function in **R**. We do this for all six principal components, for five principal components, and for four principal components.

```
@ Dispar6pc <- dist(BAMBISpc,method="euclidean")
@ Dispar5pc <- dist(BAMBISpc[,1:5],method="euclidean")
@ Dispar4pc <- dist(BAMBISpc[,1:4],method="euclidean")
```

We then proceed to do the corresponding hierarchical clustering operations using the `hclust()` facility of **R** which starts with individual cases and merges mergers into progressively larger collectives.

```
@ ClusPC6 <- hclust(Dispar6pc,method="ward")
@ ClusPC5 <- hclust(Dispar5pc,method="ward")
@ ClusPC4 <- hclust(Dispar4pc,method="ward")
```

We plot the respective clustering dendrograms which give a visualization of how the clustering has transpired (Figs. 4.1–4.3).

```
@ plot(ClusPC6,labels=F)
```

Since some structural differences appear between clustering five components in Fig. 4.2 and clustering four in Fig. 4.3, preference is to retain all but the last PC-axis.

```
@ plot(ClusPC5,labels=F)
@ plot(ClusPC4,labels=F)
```

Cutting Clusters

The next task is to decide how many collectives should be differentiated. In preparation for this, it is helpful to know the attributes of an output from `hclust()`.

```
@ attributes(ClusPC6)
$names
[1] "merge"        "height"      "order"       "labels"      "method"
[6] "call"         "dist.method"
```

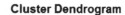

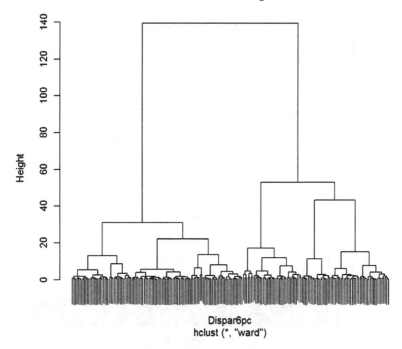

Fig. 4.1 Dendrogram from clustering all six BAMBISpc principal components

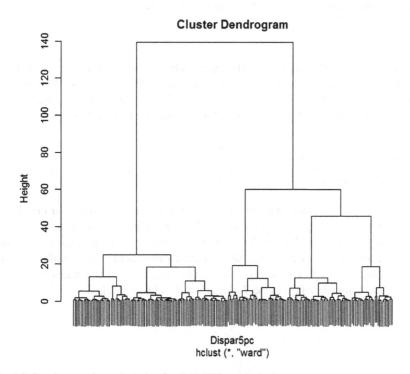

Fig. 4.2 Dendrogram from clustering five BAMBISpc principal components

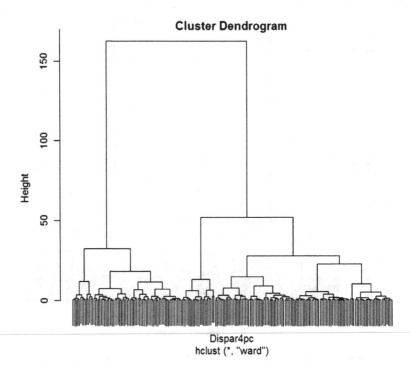

Fig. 4.3 Dendrogram from clustering four BAMBISpc principal components

The heights give the disparities (linkages) between the collectives being merged and the later mergers are at the top of the dendrogram. Therefore, it is informative to have a reversed listing of the heights and to plot the first part of the reversed listing (Fig. 4.4). This is intuitively analogous to a screeplot for principal components.

```
@ Nstep <- length(ClusPC5$height)
@ ClusPC5hts <- rep(0,Nstep)
@ for(I in 1:Nstep) ClusPC5hts[I] <- ClusPC5$height[Nstep - I +1]
@ plot(ClusPC5hts[1:25])
```

The top bar (partition/point) entails two clusters, and each lower bar entails an additional cluster. Thus, Fig. 4.4 shows that there are definitely five clusters followed by another somewhat elevated level of three additional clusters, then a second relatively level set of three more clusters with a subsequent gradual trailing off of slight changes in level. To encompass a span in this progression, we determine and cross-tabulate memberships at the 7-cluster and 12-cluster levels using cutree().

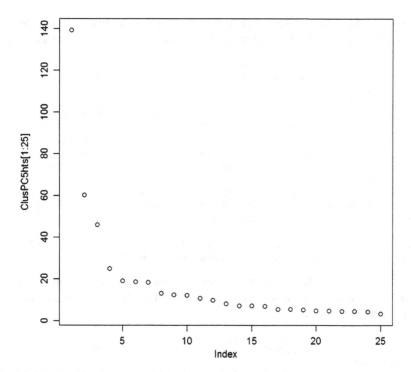

Fig. 4.4 Heights of last 25 mergers in dendrogram for clustering five principal components

```
@ Hclus7 <- cutree(ClusPC5,k=7)
@ Hclus12 <- cutree(ClusPC5,k=12)
@ Xtab12x7 <- table(Hclus12,Hclus7)
@ Xtab12x7
        Hclus7
Hclus12  1   2   3   4   5   6   7
      1  7   0   0   0   0   0   0
      2  0  12   0   0   0   0   0
      3  0   0  15   0   0   0   0
      4  0   0   0  11   0   0   0
      5  0   0   0   0  25   0   0
      6  0   0   0  31   0   0   0
      7  0   0   0   0   0  16   0
      8  0   0   0   0  13   0   0
      9  0   0   0   0   0   0  19
     10  0   0   0  22   0   0   0
     11  0   0   0   0   0  27   0
     12  0   0   0   0   0   0  13
```

Since clusters 4, 5, 6, and 7 become large as a result of the additional aggregations, the finer breakdown into 12 collectives will be at least provisionally retained. In order to proceed with the comparatives, the averages (centroids) for the provisional clusters are determined. It is also time to begin reconnecting with the original scales of measurement, so we determine centroids first for original scales, then for standardized scales, and also for principal component scales using all components.

```
@ Centr12 <- matrix(rep(0.0,72),ncol=6)
@ for(I in 1:12) Centr12[I,] <- mean(BAMBIV[Hclus12==I,])
@ Centr12
             [,1]      [,2]       [,3]      [,4]      [,5]       [,6]
 [1,]    77.57143 37.71429  20.14286 26.74286 17.32857  56.671429
 [2,]    98.50000 38.58333  39.00000 91.76667 90.95833   2.866667
 [3,]   114.53333 38.93333  36.13333 59.12000 49.78000  21.553333
 [4,]   109.45455 46.63636  73.00000 90.38182 86.35455   4.736364
 [5,]   128.24000 48.64000 111.88000 92.90000 92.59600   2.444000
 [6,]   132.51613 48.35484  64.58065 89.72258 89.17742   3.406452
 [7,]   130.06250 43.50000  72.37500 53.62500 43.96875  26.900000
 [8,]   125.46154 48.69231 151.92308 78.87692 71.46154  10.838462
 [9,]   118.31579 42.63158  39.31579 42.36316 24.38947  40.584211
[10,]   126.54545 45.36364  93.04545 77.10000 74.84091   8.959091
[11,]   129.51852 48.25926  74.29630 64.89630 56.08519  16.670370
[12,]   120.84615 42.30769  46.15385 26.81538 11.00769  69.115385
```

With the Centr12 object containing centroids on original scales, we use Centr12S as the object designation for standardized scales and Centr12PC as the designation for principal components.

```
@ Centr12S <- matrix(rep(0.0,72),ncol=6)
@ for(I in 1:12) Centr12S[I,] <- mean(BAMBIS[Hclus12==I,])
@ round(Centr12S,6)
             [,1]       [,2]       [,3]       [,4]       [,5]       [,6]
 [1,]   -3.001888  -1.787566  -1.416603  -1.912644  -1.622231   1.889115
 [2,]   -1.592476  -1.578957  -0.905863   0.966024   0.967379  -0.759819
 [3,]   -0.512729  -1.494942  -0.983506  -0.479276  -0.480892   0.160169
 [4,]   -0.854754   0.354118   0.015019   0.904715   0.805460  -0.667769
 [5,]    0.410332   0.835077   1.068073   1.016197   1.024976  -0.780628
 [6,]    0.698303   0.766626  -0.213017   0.875530   0.904743  -0.733244
 [7,]    0.533066  -0.398745  -0.001909  -0.722545  -0.685277   0.423398
 [8,]    0.223219   0.847633   2.152630   0.395382   0.281663  -0.367349
 [9,]   -0.258003  -0.607203  -0.897310  -1.221118  -1.373894   1.097103
[10,]    0.296215   0.048608   0.557944   0.316716   0.400518  -0.459875
[11,]    0.496432   0.743683   0.050128  -0.223554  -0.259134  -0.080230
[12,]   -0.087599  -0.684950  -0.712103  -1.909433  -1.844540   2.501759
```

```
@ Centr12PC <- matrix(rep(0.0,72),ncol=6)
@ for(I in 1:12) Centr12PC[I,] <- mean(BAMBISpc[Hclus12==I,])
@ round(Centr12PC,6)
             [,1]       [,2]       [,3]       [,4]       [,5]       [,6]
 [1,]   -4.495382  -1.479531   1.143377  -0.674915   0.009665  -0.162243
 [2,]   -0.040095  -2.862384  -0.111296   0.332022   0.112365   0.073655
 [3,]   -1.579076  -0.963333  -0.438824   0.557360  -0.212756   0.022029
 [4,]    1.058017  -1.121738   0.292976  -0.556565   0.054630   0.079546
 [5,]    2.135544   0.097771   0.355831   0.042200   0.151176  -0.011762
 [6,]    1.583769  -0.070853  -0.797950  -0.288761   0.159217  -0.011064
 [7,]   -0.891760   0.734332  -0.158155   0.483995  -0.161868  -0.042935
 [8,]    1.631199   0.901789   1.489003   0.304788  -0.124310   0.026632
 [9,]   -2.361537   0.430415  -0.207175  -0.134082  -0.127853   0.105568
[10,]    0.844000   0.024319   0.137789   0.366812  -0.078706  -0.071538
[11,]    0.232101   0.799563  -0.199419  -0.368185  -0.246994  -0.022061
[12,]   -3.491662   1.344071   0.153459  -0.068377   0.576518   0.014450
```

It will also be helpful to have a vector object of hexagon ID numbers for identifying which hexagons have membership in each collective.

```
@ HexNmbrs <- BAMBI[,1]
```

Comparing Cluster Collectives

Having at least provisionally reduced the scope of study from 211 hexagons to 12 collectives, we proceed to make scatter plots for centroids in terms of pairs of original BAMBIV variates (Fig. 4.5). The intent is to see if the centroids capture important aspects of relationships contained in the original data.

```
@ pairs(Centr12)
```

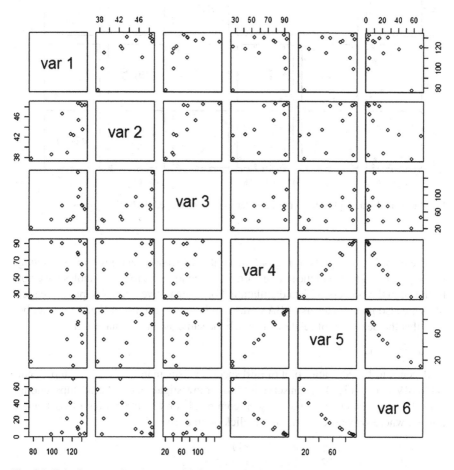

Fig. 4.5 Paired scatter plots for centroids in terms of original BAMBIV variates

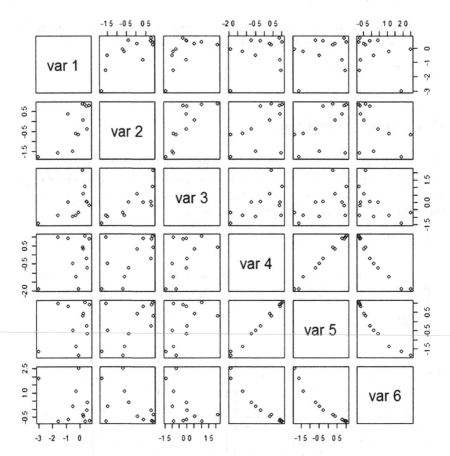

Fig. 4.6 Paired scatter plots for centroids in terms of standardized BAMBIS variates

The paired scatter plots of Fig. 4.5 make the dispersions and proximities among the centroids evident, and the strong correlations among the forest variables have not been lost in the process of data distillation. For comparative purposes, paired scatter plots are also given in terms of BAMBIS standardized variates in Fig. 4.6. It can be seen that the depiction of relations is much the same as for original variates.

```
@ pairs(Centr12S)
```

A centroid-based scatter plot of bird species versus mammal species on original BAMBIV scales (Fig. 4.7) can serve for further investigation of relationships among collectives by using the `identify()` command for tagging things of particular interest whereby we use the mouse to click on interesting items.

```
@ plot(Centr12[,1],Centr12[,2])
@ identify(Centr12[,1],Centr12[,2])
```

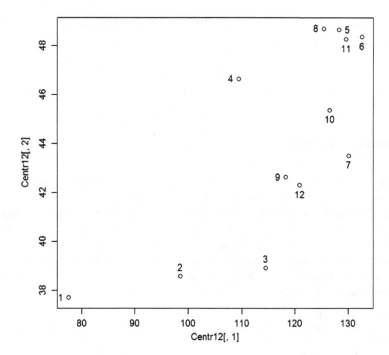

Fig. 4.7 Centroid-based scatter plot of bird species (*horizontal*) versus mammal species (*vertical*) on original BAMBIV scales

The hexagons having membership in collective 1 that occupies the lowest position on both axes can be determined as follows:

```
@ HexNmbrs[Hclus12==1]
[1] 1714 1829 2294 2296 2415 4306 4312
```

Thus, the collective numbered one is impoverished with regard to habitat richness for both birds and also for mammals. The first five of these are hexagons situated in the heavily urbanized and agricultural areas of southeastern Pennsylvania. The remaining two hexagons are likewise in areas that are heavily impacted by human habitation.

The hexagon memberships of collectives having high species richness can be similarly determined.

```
@ HexNmbrs[Hclus12==5]
 [1] 2054 2171 2286 2527 2647 2648 2770 2891 2892 2894 2895 2897 3017 3021 3022
[16] 3141 3142 3143 3267 3268 3274 3394 3395 3529 3778
@ HexNmbrs[Hclus12==6]
 [1] 2055 2170 2287 2288 2289 2290 2405 2525 2526 2528 2646 2769 3014 3015 3016
[16] 3140 3265 3266 3392 3393 3520 3521 3522 3649 3650 3651 3781 3910 3911 4042
[31] 4043
@ HexNmbrs[Hclus12==8]
 [1] 2172 2404 2408 2524 2645 2893 3271 3272 3273 3275 3527 3528 3658
@ HexNmbrs[Hclus12==11]
 [1] 2292 2407 2649 2650 2651 2771 3019 3020 3144 3145 3146 3147 3269 3396 3397
[16] 3398 3399 3400 3401 3523 3524 3526 3652 3909 3912 4041 4044
```

Also interesting are collectives 2 and 3 which have low mammal species richness but moderate bird species richness.

```
@ HexNmbrs[Hclus12==2]
 [1] 1827 1941 2058 2059 2060 2061 3402 3788 3918 3919 4049 4050
@ HexNmbrs[Hclus12==3]
 [1] 1828 1942 1943 1944 2057 2176 2178 2293 2414 2533 3786 3787 4180 4442 4444
```

Exploring Exchange

The early mergers in the hierarchical strategy somewhat constrain the combinations of cases (hexagons) that can appear in the later collectives of clusters (Basu et al. 2009). Thus, additional insight can be obtained by revisiting the clusters through a different strategy called *kmeans* that permits cluster adjustment by exchanges (Gan et al. 2007). This strategy operates directly on a data matrix of case measures instead of (dis)similarities, and needs a set of tentative positions around which to organize clusters for subsequent adjustment. We will use the data on the first five principal components, and start from hierarchical clusters.

```
@ KdataPC5 <- BAMBISpc[,1:5]
@ KstartPC5 <- Centr12PC[,1:5]
@ Kmeans12PC <- kmeans(KdataPC5,KstartPC5)
@ attributes(Kmeans12PC)
$names
[1] "cluster" "centers"  "withinss" "size"

$class
[1] "kmeans"
```

As with the previous comparison of 12 hierarchical clusters with 7 hierarchical clusters, our primary way of cluster comparison is by cross-tabulation of clusterings in terms of member cases.

```
@ Klus12 <- Kmeans12PC$cluster
@ Klus12siz <- Kmeans12PC$size
@ XtabHxK <- table(Klus12,Hclus12)
@ XtabHxK
       Hclus12
Klus12   1  2  3  4  5  6  7  8  9 10 11 12
     1   6  0  0  0  0  0  0  0  0  0  0  0
     2   0 11  0  0  0  0  0  0  0  1  0  0
     3   0  0 12  0  0  0  0  0  0  1  0  0
     4   0  1  0  5  0  0  0  0  0  0  0  0
     5   0  0  0  0 25  2  0  0  0  0  0  0
     6   0  0  0  5  0 29  0  0  0  0  0  0
     7   0  0  0  0  0  0 16  0  0  0  3  0
     8   0  0  0  0  0  0  0 13  0  3  1  0
     9   1  0  3  0  0  0  0  0 19  0  0  0
    10   0  0  0  1  0  0  0  0  0 17  0  0
    11   0  0  0  0  0  0  0  0  0  0 23  0
    12   0  0  0  0  0  0  0  0  0  0  0 13
```

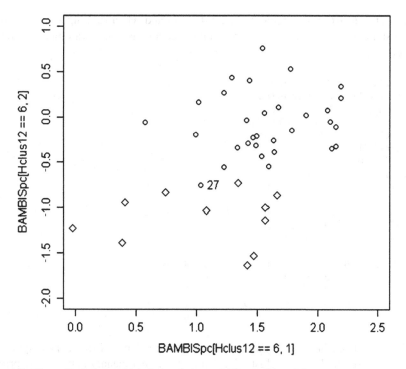

Fig. 4.8 Hierarchical cluster 6 (*circles*) and cluster 4 (*diamonds*) on PC axes 1 and 2

This shows high consistency, with 189 of the 211 hexagons retaining their membership. It is notable, however, that 5 of the 11 members in cluster four have shifted to cluster six. This leaves cluster 4 with only 6 members, and hierarchical cluster 4 and cluster 6 show considerable disparity of position in Fig. 4.7. Thus, it is appropriate to examine the positioning of members within hierarchical clusters 4 and 6 in terms of the first two PC axes using different symbols (plotting characters) as shown in Fig. 4.8, with circles for cluster 6 and diamonds for cluster 4.

```
@ plot(BAMBISpc[Hclus12==6,1],BAMBISpc[Hclus12==6,2],
@@ xlim=c(0.0,2.5),ylim=c(-2.0,1.0))
@ points(BAMBISpc[Hclus12==4,1],BAMBISpc[Hclus12==4,2],pch=5)
@ identify(BAMBISpc[Hclus12==6,1],BAMBISpc[Hclus12==6,2])
```

Figure 4.8 shows that hierarchical clusters 4 and 6 are reasonably well separated on principal component axis 2, except for case number 27. However, it also shows that cluster 4 spreads widely and lacks compactness of shape. Since *kmeans* favors compactness more so than *hclust*, it would have a propensity to pull this kind of hierarchical cluster apart. Therefore, it is reasonable to see what happens if the centroid from hierarchical cluster 4 is deleted when running *kmeans*. The 11 clusters that result can then be cross-tabulated against the hierarchical clusters as before.

```
@ KstrtPC5 <- KstartPC5[-4,]
@ Kmeans11PC <- kmeans(KdataPC5,KstrtPC5)
@ Klus11 <- Kmeans11PC$cluster
@ Klus11siz <- Kmeans11PC$size
@ XtabHxK11 <- table(Klus11, Hclus12)
@ XtabHxK11
       Hclus12
Klus11  1  2  3  4  5  6  7  8  9 10 11 12
     1  6  0  0  0  0  0  0  0  0  0  0  0
     2  0 11  0  0  0  0  0  0  0  0  0  0
     3  0  1 12  0  0  0  0  0  0  1  0  0
     4  0  0  0  0 25  2  0  0  0  0  0  0
     5  0  0  0  4  0 29  0  0  0  0  0  0
     6  0  0  0  0  0  0 16  0  0  0  3  0
     7  0  0  0  0  0  0  0 13  0  4  0  0
     8  1  0  3  0  0  0  0  0 19  0  0  0
     9  0  0  0  7  0  0  0  0  0 15  2  0
    10  0  0  0  0  0  0  0  0  0  2 22  0
    11  0  0  0  0  0  0  0  0  0  0  0 13
```

The 11 clusters produced by *kmeans* have a better balance of sizes, and it appears that the questionable fourth cluster has been split rather cleanly between the prior cluster 6 (which has become cluster 5) and prior cluster 10 (which has become cluster 9). Accordingly, centroids are recalculated for the 11 collectives from *kmeans*, this time including centroids from rank rescaling. Each of these collectives will now be called a *contingent* since they arise from comparative and complementary clustering methodologies, including cross-tabulations in the manner of contingency tables.

```
@ Centr11 <- matrix(rep(0.0,66),ncol=6)
@ for(I in 1:11) Centr11[I,] <- mean(BAMBIV[Klus11==I,])
@ Centr11
           [,1]      [,2]       [,3]      [,4]      [,5]        [,6]
[1,]   73.33333 37.50000  21.00000 29.21667 18.85000 58.383333
[2,]   96.72727 38.72727  38.81818 92.72727 92.22727  2.654545
[3,]  116.21429 38.71429  37.57143 63.23571 56.62143 17.885714
[4,]  128.88889 48.66667 110.44444 92.71481 92.41481  2.618519
[5,]  130.39394 48.24242  62.15152 90.41212 89.91212  3.233333
[6,]  130.94737 44.05263  74.78947 53.43158 43.86842 27.931579
```

```
 [7,]  125.70588 48.58824 143.41176 77.97647 71.78824 10.664706
 [8,]  116.73913 42.08696  38.08696 41.69565 24.37826 39.326087
 [9,]  118.70833 45.33333  86.00000 80.63750 77.20000  7.570833
[10,]  130.37500 48.37500  73.95833 66.97500 58.14583 14.887500
[11,]  120.84615 42.30769  46.15385 26.81538 11.00769 69.115385

@ Centr11S <- matrix(rep(0.0,66),ncol=6)
@ for(I in 1:11) Centr11S[I,] <- mean(BAMBIS[Klus11==I,])
@ round(Centr11S,6)
            [,1]       [,2]       [,3]       [,4]       [,5]       [,6]
 [1,] -3.287298 -1.839004 -1.393388 -1.803126 -1.568721  1.973396
 [2,] -1.711858 -1.544405 -0.910787  1.008551  1.012008 -0.770262
 [3,] -0.399527 -1.547523 -0.944555 -0.297070 -0.240274 -0.020396
 [4,]  0.454031  0.841478  1.029192  1.007999  1.018604 -0.772036
 [5,]  0.555387  0.739642 -0.278810  0.906057  0.930583 -0.741767
 [6,]  0.592657 -0.266089  0.063486 -0.731108 -0.688806  0.474185
 [7,]  0.239674  0.822652  1.922103  0.355518  0.293153 -0.375903
 [8,] -0.364182 -0.737936 -0.930592 -1.250669 -1.374288  1.035163
 [9,] -0.231568  0.041334  0.367120  0.473324  0.483489 -0.528222
[10,]  0.554111  0.771466  0.040975 -0.131528 -0.186660 -0.168005
[11,] -0.087599 -0.684950 -0.712103 -1.909433 -1.844540  2.501759

@ Centr11PC <- matrix(rep(0.0,66),ncol=6)
@ for(I in 1:11) Centr11PC[I,] <- mean(BAMBISpc[Klus11==I,])
@ round(Centr11PC,6)
            [,1]       [,2]       [,3]       [,4]       [,5]       [,6]
 [1,] -4.538416 -1.703134  1.329765 -0.752994  0.117290 -0.108933
 [2,] -0.011606 -2.955142 -0.051756  0.252962  0.128507  0.073778
 [3,] -1.271773 -1.092869 -0.538077  0.691055 -0.176431 -0.012714
 [4,]  2.124193  0.122813  0.302320  0.039901  0.157205 -0.012321
 [5,]  1.545884 -0.215538 -0.772466 -0.353390  0.166348 -0.004977
 [6,] -0.832572  0.871907 -0.126797  0.424306 -0.126791 -0.047090
 [7,]  1.534846  0.831715  1.297073  0.242305 -0.128143 -0.007249
 [8,] -2.435370  0.284581 -0.184895 -0.083588 -0.191262  0.081908
 [9,]  0.790274 -0.471369  0.268704  0.077394 -0.078876 -0.014270
[10,]  0.373359  0.767147 -0.265827 -0.357579 -0.249855 -0.008097
[11,] -3.491662  1.344071  0.153459 -0.068377  0.576518  0.014450

@ Centr11R <- matrix(rep(0.0,66),ncol=6)
@ for(I in 1:11) Centr11R[I,] <- mean(BAMBIR[Klus11==I,])
@ round(Centr11R,6)
            [,1]       [,2]       [,3]       [,4]       [,5]       [,6]
 [1,]   5.083333  18.50000   7.333333  16.33333  21.66667 192.00000
 [2,]  19.863636  23.36364  42.409091 176.00000 176.45454  38.72727
 [3,]  61.392857  22.85714  43.857143  76.14286  80.35714 127.21429
 [4,] 134.370370 161.50000 174.148148 174.87037 175.75926  37.83333
 [5,] 148.106061 155.03030  95.833333 165.33333 167.25758  47.27273
 [6,] 144.842105  76.97368 115.052632  52.55263  57.84210 158.34211
 [7,] 121.617647 159.35294 197.705882 121.67647 115.02941  98.02941
 [8,]  62.021739  58.28261  43.956522  30.23913  28.78261 177.21739
 [9,]  80.604167  96.04167 138.166667 129.64583 127.50000  86.33333
[10,] 141.416667 152.31250 115.375000  85.18750  81.60417 123.72917
[11,]  89.807692  56.07692  56.461538  13.07692  13.07692 202.53846
```

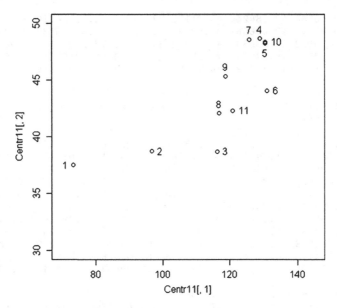

Fig. 4.9 Centroid-based scatter plot of bird species (*horizontal*) versus mammal species (*vertical*) on original BAMBIV scales for 11 contingents

Since interpretation is often most easily done in terms of the original scales of measurement, we first make a plot of the centroids for the 11 contingents relative to birds (X) and mammals (Y) as was done previously for 12 hierarchical clusters in Fig. 4.7. This scatter plot with ID numbers for the contingents is in Fig. 4.9.

```
@ plot(Centr11[,1],Centr11[,2],xlim=c(70,145),ylim=c(30,50))
@ identify(Centr11[,1],Centr11[,2])
```

Contingents 1 and 2 are low whereas 4, 5, 7, and 10 are high. Since contingents 5 and 10 are almost the same with respect to the biodiversity variates, we also need paired scatter plots to see the situation with respect to other habitat variates (Fig. 4.10).

```
@ pairs(Centr11)
```

At least in terms of the relationship of topographic variability (variate 3) to variates for forest cover (variates 4, 5, and 6), the contingents are quite well spread. To finalize the construction of contingents, we first cast the centroids as data frames, and provide variate names and then replot Fig. 4.10 with variate names as Fig. 4.11.

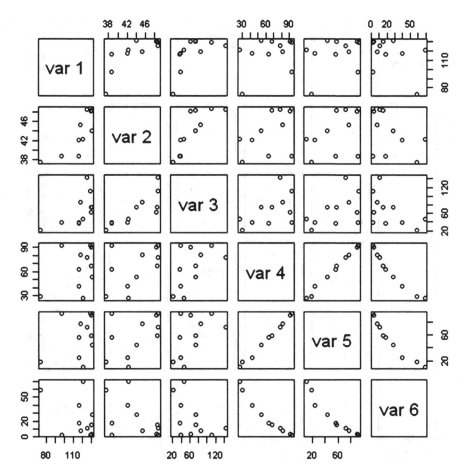

Fig. 4.10 Paired scatter plots for contingents in terms of original BAMBIV variates

```
@ Centr11 <- as.data.frame(Centr11)
@ Centr11S <- as.data.frame(Centr11S)
@ Centr11PC <- as.data.frame(Centr11PC)
@ Centr11R <- as.data.frame(Centr11R)
@ names(Centr11) <- c("BirdSp","MamlSp","ElevSD","PctFor",
@@ "Pct1FPch","Pct1OPch")
@ names(Centr11S) <- c("BirdSp","MamlSp","ElevSD","PctFor",
@@ "Pct1FPch","Pct1OPch")
@ names(Centr11PC) <- c("BirdSp","MamlSp","ElevSD","PctFor",
@@ "Pct1FPch","Pct1OPch")
@ names(Centr11R) <- c("BirdSp","MamlSp","ElevSD","PctFor",
@@ "Pct1FPch","Pct1OPch")
@ pairs(Centr11)
```

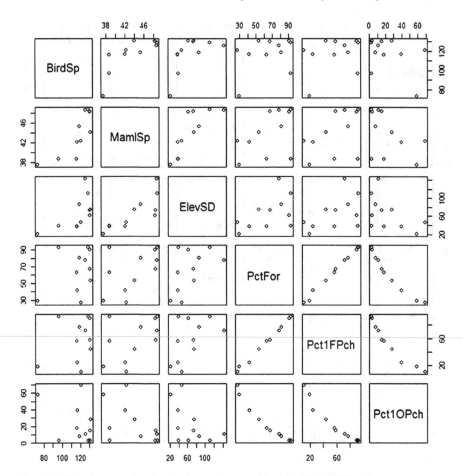

Fig. 4.11 Paired scatter plots for contingents in terms of original BAMBIV variates

The column of memberships for contingents is bound together with the column of hexagon IDs and cast as data frame then written to a file. Files are also written for selected other data frames. Hexagon memberships of contingents are then listed.

```
@ CONTINGN <- cbind(HexNmbrs,Klus11)
@ CONTINGN <- as.data.frame(CONTINGN)
@ write.table(CONTINGN,"Contingn.txt",row.names=F)
@ write.table(BAMBIS,"BAMBIs.txt",row.names=F)
@ write.table(BAMBISpc,"BAMBIspc.txt",row.names=F)
```

```
@ write.table(BAMBIR,"BAMBIrnk.txt",row.names=F)
@ write.table(Centrll,"Centrll.txt",row.names=F)
@ write.table(CentrllS,"Centrlls.txt",row.names=F)
@ write.table(CentrllPC,"Cntrllpc.txt",row.names=F)
@ write.table(CentrllR,"Cntrllr.txt",row.names=F)
@ HexNmbrs[Klus11==1]
[1] 1714 1829 2296 2415 4306 4312
@ HexNmbrs[Klus11==2]
 [1] 1827 1941 2059 2060 2061 3402 3788 3918 3919 4049 4050
@ HexNmbrs[Klus11==3]
 [1] 1828 1942 1943 1944 2057 2058 2176 2178 2293 2295 2533 3787 4180
4444
@ HexNmbrs[Klus11==4]
 [1] 2054 2171 2286 2290 2527 2647 2648 2770 2891 2892 2894 2895 2897
3017 3021
[16] 3022 3140 3141 3142 3143 3267 3268 3274 3394 3395 3529 3778
@ HexNmbrs[Klus11==5]
 [1] 2055 2169 2170 2287 2288 2289 2405 2525 2526 2528 2646 2767 2769
3014 3015
[16] 3016 3265 3266 3392 3393 3520 3521 3522 3649 3650 3651 3779 3780
3781 3910
[31] 3911 4042 4043
@ HexNmbrs[Klus11==6]
 [1] 2056 2173 2292 2407 2411 2532 2653 2771 2772 2775 2776 2899 2900
3657 3783
[16] 3784 3913 4175 4309
@ HexNmbrs[Klus11==7]
 [1] 2172 2404 2408 2524 2645 2893 2896 2898 3018 3270 3271 3272 3273
3275 3527
[16] 3528 3658
@ HexNmbrs[Klus11==8]
 [1] 2174 2177 2294 2412 2413 2414 2534 3525 3653 3654 3655 3782 3786
3917 4047
[16] 4048 4173 4174 4179 4308 4310 4442 4443
@ HexNmbrs[Klus11==9]
 [1] 2053 2175 2406 2409 2410 2529 2530 2531 2650 2652 2654 2655 2773
2774 2890
[16] 3023 3024 3139 3148 3149 3391 3396 3519 3648
@ HexNmbrs[Klus11==10]
 [1] 2291 2649 2651 2768 3019 3020 3144 3145 3146 3147 3269 3397 3398
3399 3400
[16] 3401 3523 3524 3526 3652 3909 3912 4041 4044
@ HexNmbrs[Klus11==11]
 [1] 2777 3656 3785 3914 3915 3916 4045 4046 4176 4177 4178 4307 4311
```

Tagging Trees

Of direct interest for many practical purposes are the distinguishing characteristics of collectives in terms of original measurements. We have not yet addressed that question for the foregoing contingents. The classification tree approach (Breiman et al. 1998; Fielding 2007; Halgamuge and Wang 2005) allows us to consider that question while making minimal assumptions about distributions of the data. This is accomplished here through the *tree* package for **R** that is available for downloading from the cooperative **CRAN** Web site associated with the **R**-project.

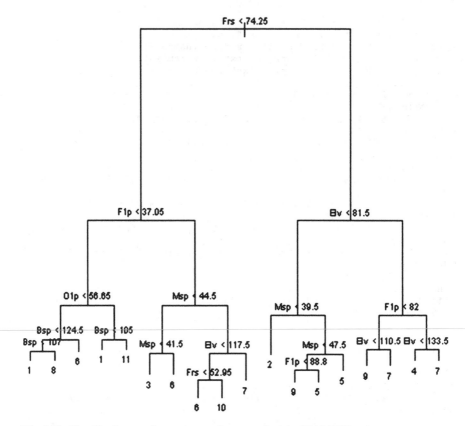

Fig. 4.12 Classification tree for contingents in terms of original BAMBIV variates

After downloading, such a package requires an initial installation through the **R** menus and then activation for each new session via the library() command in **R**.

The classification tree is a kind of modeling operation, and it requires that categorization be declared as what **R** calls a *factor* with a specific number of levels. Since the tree is depicted graphically, it is also important to use short labels for the variates involved. A command sequence to obtain a tree is as follows, with the tree being shown in Fig. 4.12.

```
@ library(tree)
@ Cntngn <- Klus11
@ Cntngn <- factor(Cntngn,levels=1:11)
@ Bsp <- BAMBIV$BirdSp
@ Msp <- BAMBIV$MamlSp
@ Elv <- BAMBIV$ElevSD
@ Frs <- BAMBIV$PctFor
@ Flp <- BAMBIV$Pct1FPch
@ Olp <- BAMBIV$Pct1OPch
@ CntngnTree <- tree(Cntngn ~ Bsp + Msp + Elv + Frs + Flp + Olp)
@ plot(CntngnTree)
@ text(CntngnTree,cex=0.6)
```

According to the classification tree model, percent forest is the single most influential variable in segregating contingents. Within one branch of the first split, the forest integrity assumes second importance, and within the other branch it is topographic variability. It is important to note that the hierarchical clustering and the kmeans clustering are both **polythetic** in that several variates are considered simultaneously. In contrast, a tree model is **monothetic** in that each successive split is based on one particular variate. The latter is important from an interpretive standpoint. The foregoing scenario allows combining the best features of polythetic and monothetic approaches.

Contingent Cartography

The file with the two-column data frame of hexagon IDs and contingent numbers can be imported into Excel for structuring and saving as a dbf file, which is then joined in a geographic information system to the table of hexagon attributes for mapping as hexagon labels to produce the map of contingents shown in Fig. 4.13. The hexagons without a contingent number in Fig. 4.13 are ones that lie outside Pennsylvania.

Computational Considerations and Characterizing Collectives

Computational constraints also arise for clustering with large numbers of cases (Mirkin 2005). The effective size of a (symmetric) distance matrix is roughly half the square for the number of cases. However, some clustering methods like k-means

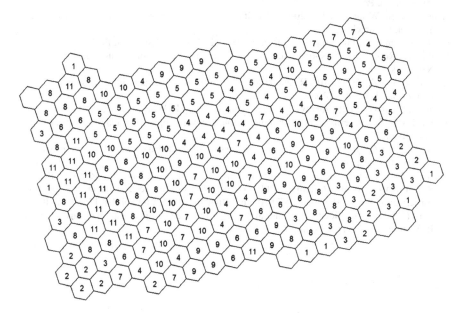

Fig. 4.13 Map of membership in contingents for hexagons in Pennsylvania

do not use case-to-case distances, and thus do not require prior computation of a distance matrix as input. Adaptations of such approaches can be used with very large data sets, such as image data in remote sensing (Myers and Patil 2006). Thus, creating collectives by clustering for preliminary prioritization is still viable but the scenario may not be as simple and straightforward as the pattern we have presented.

Performing preliminary prioritization on collectives from clustering will require characterizing the clusters by assigning attributes that serve as collective criteria. Centroids are commonly used in clustering contexts, so that is how we have cast collective characteristics up to this point. This is by no means even the primary possibility, but it provides a point of departure for paths to this end in the next chapter. Collateral considerations include reducing the dimensionality for displays and exploring alternatives to averaging over the aggregates that is at the essence of constructing centroids.

References

Abonyi J, Balaz F (2007) Cluster analysis for data mining and system identification. Birkhauser, Berlin

Basu S, Davidson I, Wagstaff K (2009) Constrained clustering: advances in algorithms, theory, and applications. Chapman & Hall/CRC, Boca Raton, FL

Breiman L, Freidman J, Olsen R, Stone C (1998) Classification and regression trees (CART). Chapman & Hall/CRC, Boca Raton, FL

Everitt B, Landau S, Leese M (2001) Cluster analysis. Arnold, London

Fielding A (2007) Cluster and classification techniques for the biosciences. Cambridge University Press, Cambridge

Gan G, Ma C, Ma C, Wu J (2007) Data clustering: theory, algorithms, and applications. SIAM, Philadelphia, PA

Halgamuge S, Wang L (eds) (2005) Classification and clustering for knowledge discovery. Springer, Dordrecht

Hardle W, Simar L (2007) Applied multivariate statistical analysis. Springer, Berlin

Kaufman L, Rousseeuw P (1990) Finding groups in data: an introduction to cluster analysis. Wiley, New York

Long B, Zhang Z, Yu P (2010) Relational data clustering: models, algorithms and applications. Chapman & Hall/CRC, Boca Raton, FL

Lumley T (2010) Complex surveys: a guide to analysis using R. Wiley, Hoboken, NJ

Mirkin B (2005) Clustering for data mining: a data recovery approach. Chapman & Hall/CRC, Boca Raton, FL

Myers W, Patil GP (2006) Pattern-based compression of multi-band image data for landscape analysis. Springer, New York

Myers W, McKenney-Easterling M, Hychka K, Griscom B, Bishop J, Bayard A, Rocco G, Brooks R, Constantz G, Patil GP, Taillie C (2006) Contextual clustering for configuring collaborative conservation of watershed in the Mid-Atlantic Highlands. Environ Ecol Stat 13(4):391–407

Podani J (2000) Introduction to the exploration of multivariate biological data. Backhuys, Leiden

Xu R, Wunsch D (2009) Clustering. Wiley, New York

Chapter 5
Distance Domains, Skeletal Structures, and Representative Ranks

Prioritization can proceed through partnership between procedures and perception. Perception is promoted by pictorial portrayal on a page, which is most manageable in two dimensions. Therefore, we consider capturing contrasts among contingents compactly in couplets of coordinates on synthetic scales (Zuur et al. 2007). What we call "distance domains" derived through multidimensional scaling are appropriate for this (Borg and Groenen 2005; Cox and Cox 2001; Green et al. 1989).

The classical version of multidimensional scaling called *principal coordinates* (PCOs) suits this scenario and is easily available in **R** as the cmdscale() function of the MASS package. It starts with distance data rather than conventional coordinates, and attempts to obtain a few axes (in this case two) that portray the distance relations to the best advantage. A preliminary is computation of distances among the instances of interest, for which we use centroids of the contingents. We do distances on both original observations and standardized scales for comparison.

```
@ Dist11 <- dist(Centr11,method="euclidean")
@ round(Dist11,2)
          1       2       3       4       5       6       7       8       9      10
2  115.71
3   79.62   52.45
4  154.16   79.14   89.18
5  130.00   42.18   54.38   48.44
6   91.63   83.76   44.61   76.40   65.38
7  159.08  112.14  109.04   42.48   84.64   80.23
8   52.41   94.68   44.44  118.35   93.67   46.91  124.91
9  122.38   56.12   56.82   33.38   31.46   50.43   58.32   87.32
10 105.06   66.59   40.54   57.63   42.82   24.02   71.91   62.36   29.89
11  55.64  126.52   78.36  140.11  122.45   66.40  138.75   37.01  112.55   87.61
@ Dist11S <- dist(Centr11S,method="euclidean")
@ round(Dist11S,2)
      1    2    3    4    5    6    7    8    9   10
2  4.99
3  4.08 2.36
4  7.01 3.76 3.77
5  6.60 3.28 3.15 1.32
6  4.88 3.92 2.07 3.11 2.81
7  6.65 4.31 3.88 1.40 2.41 2.76
```

W.L. Myers and G.P. Patil, *Multivariate Methods of Representing Relations in R for Prioritization Purposes*, Environmental and Ecological Statistics 6, DOI 10.1007/978-1-4614-3122-0_5, © Springer Science+Business Media, LLC 2012

```
8   3.35 4.07 1.99 4.59 4.07 1.78 4.28
9   5.62 2.64 2.38 1.48 1.40 2.17 1.82 3.34
10  5.74 3.81 2.70 2.03 1.66 1.45 2.04 2.86 1.48
11  3.52 5.55 3.53 5.75 5.36 2.84 5.22 1.71 4.69 4.02
```

Contingent Coordinates in Distance Domains

The MASS package comes with **R**, but it must still be loaded with the library() command. It is also the second thing we have encountered that uses capital letters in an **R** name. The name *cmdscale* stands for *classical multidimensional scaling*.

```
@ library(MASS)
@ PCO11 <- cmdscale(Dist11)
@ PCO11
              [,1]          [,2]
 [1,]    85.258738   -8.731896
 [2,]   -19.021173  -55.706080
 [3,]    16.144474  -22.847221
 [4,]   -66.112967    7.428837
 [5,]   -36.580981  -26.615366
 [6,]     7.300127   20.791998
 [7,]   -63.338822   47.007291
 [8,]    50.945246    4.346180
 [9,]   -34.809140   -2.314776
[10,]   -11.277120    6.338854
[11,]    71.491618   30.302178

@ PCO11S <- cmdscale(Dist11S)
@ PCO11S
              [,1]          [,2]
 [1,]    4.1958177   1.11539315
 [2,]   -0.3177547   2.78904408
 [3,]    0.6917770   0.83450113
 [4,]   -2.6746710  -0.07931048
 [5,]   -2.1239898   0.20235420
 [6,]    0.1220914  -1.08294311
 [7,]   -2.1077209  -0.83534320
 [8,]    1.7824982  -0.65097633
 [9,]   -1.3123302   0.39225288
[10,]   -1.0314893  -0.87888432
[11,]    2.7757717  -1.80607800
```

The principal coordinates are obviously quite different between distances based on scales for original observations versus distances based on standardized scales. However, plotting is required to see whether the *patterns* in PCO space are similar or different. Deriving PCO from distance based on original data is shown in Fig. 5.1.

```
@ plot(PCO11)
@ identify(PCO11)
```

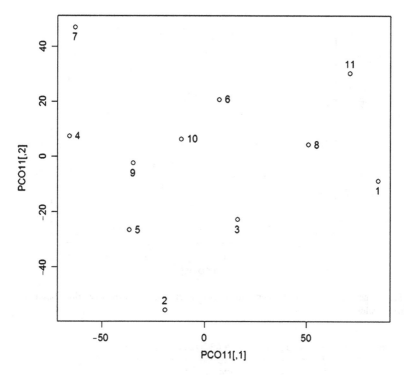

Fig. 5.1 Principal coordinates for centroids of contingents derived from disparities based on original variates

A first thing to observe in the PCO plot of Fig. 5.1 is reversal of sign sense. As with principal components, the sense of positive and negative ends of an axis is essentially indefinite. Contingent 1 has low biodiversity and contingent 7 has relatively high biodiversity. Therefore, the horizontal axis should be reversed in Fig. 5.1. To resolve the inconsistency, the principal coordinates are cast as data frames and signs changed accordingly.

Deriving PCO from distance with standardized scaling is shown in Fig. 5.2, with both axes needing to be reversed.

```
@ plot(PCO11S)
@ identify(PCO11S)
```

The required reversal based on original observations is accomplished as follows.

```
@ PCOcntr11 <- as.data.frame(PCO11)
@ PCOcntr11[,1] <- -1.0 * PCOcntr11[,1]
```

The required reversals based on standardized data are done similarly.

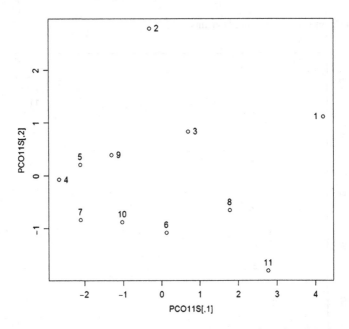

Fig. 5.2 Principal coordinates for centroids of contingents derived from disparities based on standardized scales

```
@ PCOcntr11S <- as.data.frame(PCO11S)
@ PCOcntr11S[,1] <- -1.0 * PCOcntr11S[,1]
@ PCOcntr11S[,2] <- -1.0 * PCOcntr11S[,2]
@ PCOcntr11
           V1          V2
1   -85.258738   -8.731896
2    19.021173  -55.706080
3   -16.144474  -22.847221
4    66.112967    7.428837
5    36.580981  -26.615366
6    -7.300127   20.791998
7    63.338822   47.007291
8   -50.945246    4.346180
9    34.809140   -2.314776
10   11.277120    6.338854
11  -71.491618   30.302178


@ PCOcntr11S
           V1           V2
1   -4.1958177  -1.11539315
2    0.3177547  -2.78903408
3   -0.6917770  -0.83450113
4    2.6746710   0.07931048
5    2.1239898  -0.20235420
6   -0.1220914   1.08294311
7    2.1077209   0.83534320
8   -1.7824982   0.65097633
9    1.3123302  -0.39225288
10   1.0314893   0.87888432
11  -2.7757717   1.80607800
```

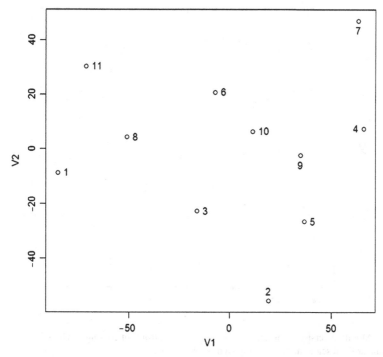

Fig. 5.3 Modified version of principal coordinates for centroids of contingents based on distances from original scales after reversing signs on first axis

The modified version of principal coordinates for centroids of contingents derived from distances based on the original scales is plotted in Fig. 5.3, and the modified version of principal coordinates for centroids of contingents derived from distances based on standardized scales is plotted in Fig. 5.4.

```
@ plot(PCOcntr11S)
@ identify(PCOcntr11S)
```

Contingents numbered 1, 2, 3, 4, 6, 8, 9, and 11 appear to be consistently placed relative to each other on either set of principal coordinates, therefore not being sensitive to scaling by standardization. The other three contingents (5, 7, 10), however, have shifted somewhat. We now seek a systematic structural screening for such scale-sensitive shifts, for which purpose we look to background concepts concerning *spanning trees* (Wu and Chao 2004).

Networks of Neighbors, Simple String Structure, and Satellite Structure

Our strategy for comparing contingents relative to scaling sensitivity entails novel notions about networks of neighbors. It satisfies our comparative criteria of being systematic, objective, and relatively straightforward. It is not necessarily the most

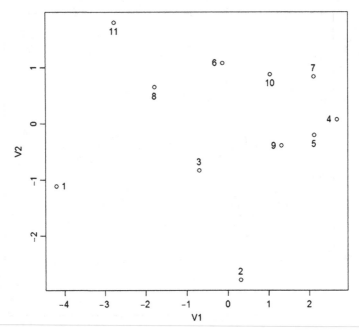

Fig. 5.4 Modified version of principal coordinates for centroids of contingents based on distances from standardized scales after reversing signs on both axes

sophisticated scenario of structures that might be conceived, but it serves to identify the contingent components that are relatively sensitive to scalings. What we do is to begin by identifying the contingent with centroid situated farthest from the origin (zero) in PCO space. This contingent becomes the anchor of a network. The linkage of the network develops progressively, whereby the (unlinked) contingent that is closest (by Euclidean distance) to any current member of the network is connected into the network by linkage to that network neighbor. The cycle is then repeated until all contingents are connected. The choice of anchor alters the nature of the network, but the anchor depends directly on disparity (distance) and defines radius of the constellation of centroids for contingents.

We formulate a *function* in **R** to perform the networking of neighbors, whereas we have thus far only used functional facilities that are already available. We call the function by the name NaborNet and list it in full detail as Function 5.1 in parallel to the way we have numbered the graphical figures. The information sent to the function is a data frame that we refer to in the function as NodeFrame. In this construct, a NodeFrame is simply a two-column listing of PCO centroids for contingents as exemplified by PCOcntr11 or PCOcntr11S. Whatever name we use to receive the function result becomes a data frame of information on the network of neighbors.

Function 5.1: NaborNet Function for Making Networks of Neighboring Centroids

```
NaborNet <- function(NodeFrame)
{
NetNode <- NodeFrame
NetNode <- NetNode[,1]
NetNode <- NetNode * 0
NetNode <- NetNode - 1
Nodes <- length(NetNode)
NetOrder <- rep(0,Nodes)
NetOrdr <- 1
Maxnode <- -1; MaxNorm <- -1
for(I in 1:Nodes)
 {VecA <- NodeFrame[I,]
  Anorm <- sum(VecA * VecA)
  if(Anorm>MaxNorm)
   {MaxNorm <- Anorm; MaxNode <- I}
 }
NetNode[MaxNode] <- MaxNode
NetOrder[MaxNode] <- NetOrdr
NetLink <- rep(0,Nodes)
LinkDist <- rep(-1,Nodes)
Undone <- Nodes-1
for(I in 1:Undone)
 {NearNode <- -1;Nearby <- -1;Nearto <- -1
  NetOrdr <- NetOrdr + 1
  for(J in 1:Nodes)
   {if(NetNode[J] < 0)
     {VecA <- NodeFrame[J,]
      for(K in 1:Nodes)
       {if(NetNode[K] > 0)
         {VecB <- NodeFrame[K,]
          VecB <- VecB - VecA
          Nearness <- sum(VecB * VecB)
          if(Nearby == -1) {NearNode<- J; Nearby<- Nearness; Nearto<- K}
          if(Nearness < Nearby) {NearNode<- J; Nearby<- Nearness; Nearto<- K}
         }
       }
     }
   }
  NetNode[NearNode] <- NearNode
  LinkDist[NearNode] <- sqrt(Nearby)
  NetLink[NearNode] <- Nearto
  NetOrder[NearNode] <- NetOrdr
  if(I == 1) {NetLink[MaxNode] <- NearNode;
   LinkDist[MaxNode] <- LinkDist[NearNode]}
 }
Nabor <- rep(1,Nodes)
for(I in 1:Nodes)
 {VecA <- NodeFrame[I,]
  for(J in 1:Nodes)
   {if(I != J)
     {VecB <- NodeFrame[J,]
      VecB <- VecB - VecA
      Nearness <- sqrt(sum(VecB * VecB))
      if(Nearness < LinkDist[I]) Nabor[I] <- Nabor[I] + 1
     }
   }
 }
Nearby <- sum(LinkDist)/Nodes
LinkDist <- LinkDist/Nearby
NetFrame <- cbind(NetNode,NetLink,NetOrder,LinkDist,Nabor)
NetFrame
}
```

For purposes of presentation, the **R** program code for NaborNet is contained in a text file called NetWorks.txt which must be incorporated into the **R** session by the source() command prior to its use. For contingents expressed in terms of original scales, this is:

```
@ source("NetWorks.txt")
@ NetFrame <- NaborNet(PCOcntr11)
@ NetFrame
        NetNode NetLink NetOrder  LinkDist Nabor
  [1,]       1       8        1 1.0911991     1
  [2,]       2       5       10 1.0097298     1
  [3,]       3       8        4 1.3124042     2
  [4,]       4       9        9 0.9742351     1
  [5,]       5       9        8 0.7240265     1
  [6,]       6      10        6 0.6994298     1
  [7,]       7       4       11 1.1789879     1
  [8,]       8       1        2 1.0911991     2
  [9,]       9      10        7 0.7450540     2
 [10,]      10       3        5 1.1900287     3
 [11,]      11       8        3 0.9837059     1
```

In a network of neighbors, the centroids of contingents are the nodes of the network. The first column of the NetFrame is contingent number as node number in the order that they occur in the NodeFrame from which the NetFrame was developed by the NaborNet function. The second column is the node (contingent) number to which it is linked in the network. The third column is the order that nodes (contingents) were linked into the network, with number 1 indicating the anchor for the network. The fourth column is the length of the link in PCO units. The fifth and final column is the order of nearness for the link node relative to the new node, with 1 indicating that a contingent is being linked to its nearest neighbor among all contingents and 2 indicating that it is linked to its second nearest neighbor among all contingents.

Representing a network graphically is a bit more complicated than most of the previous plotting scenarios.

```
@ plot(PCOcntr11)
@ Nodes <- length(NetFrame[,1])
@ for(I in 1:Nodes)
@@ {J <- NetFrame[I,1]
@@  K <- NetFrame[I,2]
@@  X <- c(PCOcntr11[J,1],PCOcntr11[K,1])
@@  Y <- c(PCOcntr11[J,2],PCOcntr11[K,2])
@@  lines(X,Y)
@@ }
@ identify(PCOcntr11)
```

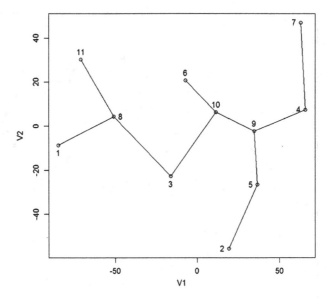

Fig. 5.5 Network of neighboring contingents for principal coordinates obtained from original scales

This plotting scenario begins with a scatterplot of the nodes as a single command, followed by a loop that plots a link in each pass after setting up the needed inputs to the lines() command which actually plots the link. One line of the NetFrame is processed in each pass. The J and K indices are first set to the respective node (contingent) number. The pair of X coordinates to be linked are then taken from the centroid frame and combined as X, and likewise for the Y coordinates. The X- and Y-pair are then fed to the lines() command, with the result as shown in Fig. 5.5.

A corresponding network of neighboring contingents is developed from principal coordinates obtained from standardized scales as follows:

```
@ NetFrameS <- NaborNet(PCOcntr11S)
@ NetFrameS
        NetNode NetLink NetOrder  LinkDist Nabor
 [1,]        1       8        1  1.8369305     1
 [2,]        2       3       11  1.3511897     1
 [3,]        3       8       10  1.1319486     1
 [4,]        4       7        7  0.5804339     2
 [5,]        5       4        8  0.3799151     1
 [6,]        6       8        4  1.0537997     2
 [7,]        7      10        6  0.6615817     3
 [8,]        8       1        2  1.8369305     5
 [9,]        9       5        9  0.5119989     1
[10,]       10       6        5  0.7195503     2
[11,]       11       8        3  0.9357210     1
```

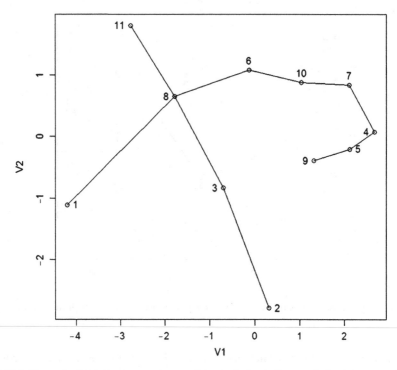

Fig. 5.6 Network of neighboring contingents for principal coordinates obtained from standardized scales

The plotting scenario for network obtained from standardized scales is the following, with the network being shown in Fig. 5.6.

```
@ plot(PCOcntr11S)
@ for(I in 1:Nodes)
@@ {J <- NetFrameS[I,1]
@@   K <- NetFrameS[I,2]
@@   X <- c(PCOcntr11S[J,1],PCOcntr11S[K,1])
@@   Y <- c(PCOcntr11S[J,2],PCOcntr11S[K,2])
@@   lines(X,Y)
@@ }
@ identify(PCOcntr11S)
```

Figure 5.6 also brings up a point regarding how the horizontal and vertical axes of the plot are graduated by default. In contrast to the situation with PCOs obtained for original scales (Fig. 5.5), the upper and lower limits for the axes are more different which gives a somewhat distorted sense of the lengths of links in the network.

The axes can be equalized by specifying the limits when the points are plotted, giving Fig. 5.7.

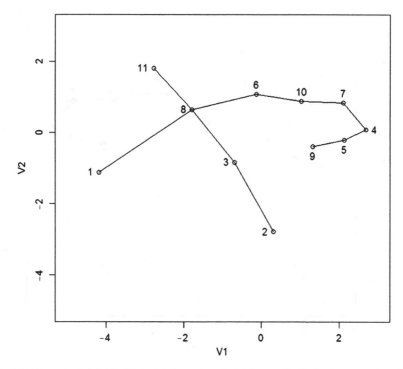

Fig. 5.7 Network of neighboring contingents for principal coordinates obtained from standardized scales as plotted on equalized axes

```
@ plot(PCOcntr11S,xlim=c(-5,3),ylim=c(-5,3))
@ for(I in 1:Nodes)
@@ {J <- NetFrameS[I,1]
@@  K <- NetFrameS[I,2]
@@  X <- c(PCOcntr11S[J,1],PCOcntr11S[K,1])
@@  Y <- c(PCOcntr11S[J,2],PCOcntr11S[K,2])
@@  lines(X,Y)
@@ }
```

The nature of the networks can now be studied comparatively between contingents expressed in terms of original scales versus standardized scales. If contingents 2, 3, and 11 were absent in Fig. 5.7, the network would have a string structure with a hook at the end opposite the anchor. Contingent 11 adds a simple stub above the string that is linked to contingent 8. Contingents 2 and 3, however, add a substantial branch in the opposite direction that is also linked to contingent 8. Contingent 8, thus, has a pivotal position in this network.

The network structure in Fig. 5.5 obtained from expressing distances on original scales has differences from those just noted for Fig. 5.7. The one derived from

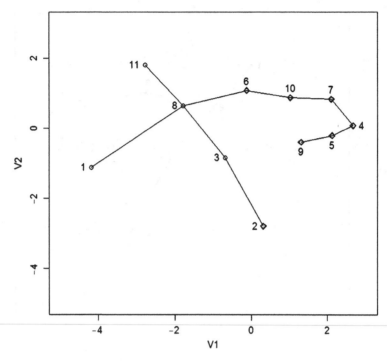

Fig. 5.8 Network of neighboring contingents for principal coordinates obtained from standardized scales, with diamonds marking nodes that link differently from original scales

original scales has a major fork at one end, a minor fork at the other, and a spur in between.

The major bifurcation is from contingent 9 and the minor one from contingent 8, with these nodes being on opposite sides of the network.

Therefore, the sense of similarities depends quite strongly upon the manner in which the contingents are expressed. The extent of the dependence can be seen more clearly by flagging the nodes that are linked differently between the two views. This requires making a node tabulation from which the contingents having the same linkage are removed, and then plotting these nodal points with a different symbol to obtain the graph in Fig. 5.8.

```
@ DiffNet <- PCOcntr11S[NetFrame[,2]!=NetFrameS[,2],]
@ points(DiffNet,pch=5)
```

Another way to examine the differences in the networks is through barplots of the linkage lengths. Of course, the large differences in PCO scales give correspondingly different vertical scales for the barplots; but it is the relative differences that are of interest. Therefore, it is appropriate to make barplots of linkages expressed as a percent of the respective maximum linkage length. A barplot of the linkage lengths based on original scales is given in Fig. 5.9, and the corresponding barplot of linkage lengths based on standardized scales is given in Fig. 5.10. It is easily seen that there

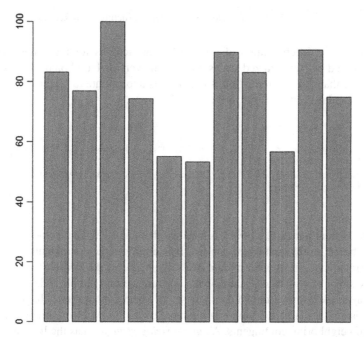

Fig. 5.9 Barplot of relative linkage lengths for network of neighboring contingents based on original scales

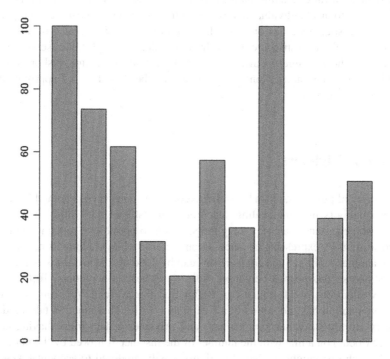

Fig. 5.10 Barplot of relative linkage lengths for network of neighboring contingents based on standardized scales

is much greater differentiation of relative linkage lengths for the version of the network based on standardized scales than for the version based on original scales. Since this enhanced differentiation is useful, it is appropriate to prefer the network having a standardized basis for further investigations.

```
@ PctLinkLngth11 <- 100.0 * (NetFrame[,4]/max(NetFrame[,4]))
@ barplot(PctLinkLngth11)
@ PctLnkLngth11S <- 100.0 * (NetFrameS[,4]/max(NetFrameS[,4]))
@ barplot(PctLnkLngth11S)
```

At the current juncture, it is well to be clear that ideas behind networks of neighbors are based on the contingent context. By definition, the contingents are few in number relative to the number of data cases. Doing networks directly for numerous data cases would most likely just give the appearance of a jumble of links, and the tabular network information would likewise pose heavy interpretive challenges.

This is also a place for summarizing some terms for types of structure in networks of neighboring contingents. A *simple string structure* has the links arranged as a string of beads so as to step sequentially through every node in order to pass from end to end. Likewise, *string structure* applies to a substantial segment of a network that is arranged in this manner, with Fig. 5.7 being illustrative in this regard. *Simple spurs* connect individual nodes into a string structure as observed in Fig. 5.5 such that the spur node has only one link. *Binary branching* is also observed in Fig. 5.5, whereby two strings emanate from a node. Although not observed in an obvious way here, a *satellite structure* would have several spurs or short strings attached to the same node. Contingent (node) number 8 in Fig. 5.7 approximates this arrangement.

k Nearest Neighbors

For a variety of purposes, it can be useful to compare an instance of something to its nearby neighbors in some scaling space or to investigate how different scalings change which instances are near neighbors. It is also possible to remain cognizant of two scalings by expressing instances in one scaling while tracking its near neighbors in another scaling. Such comparisons can be done for the nearest neighbor, for the first and second nearest neighbor, or for the *k* nearest neighbors. To facilitate such investigations, we formulate an **R** function that we call *Naboring* which is listed as Function 5.2 and stored in a NearNabr.txt file. This function takes a data frame of coordinate values as an input, and produces a data frame having each instance (locus) on a line with the number of the instance followed by the numbers of its four closest neighbors. The function is easily modified to account for more neighbors by changing the value of **K** in the function.

Function 5.2: Naboring Function for Determining *k* Nearest Neighbors

```
Naboring <- function(Loc8d)
{
Loci <- length(Loc8d[,1])
K <- 4; J <- K - 1
Locus <- seq(1:Loci); Nabor <- rep(0,Loci)
Nabors <- cbind(Locus,Nabor)
for(I in 1:J) Nabors <- cbind(Nabors,Nabor)
for(I in 1:K)
 {for(J in 1:Loci)
   {NearOne <- -1;Nearby <- -1
    VecA <- Loc8d[J,]
    for(L in 1:Loci)
     {VecB <- Loc8d[L,]
      VecB <- VecB - VecA
      Nearness <- sum(VecB * VecB)
      NotSo <- 0
      for(M in 1:I) if(Nabors[J,M] == L) NotSo <- 1
      if(NotSo == 0 & Nearby < 0)
       {NearOne <- L; Nearby <- Nearness}
      if(NotSo == 0 & Nearness < Nearby)
       {NearOne <- L; Nearby <- Nearness}
     }
    N <- I + 1; Nabors[J,N] <- NearOne
   }
 }
Nabors
}
```

As applied to the contingents expressed in principal coordinates obtained from standardized scales, the neighbor status is as follows:

```
@ source("NearNabr.txt")
@ NaborS <- Naboring(PCOcntr11S)
@ NaborS
        Locus Nabor Nabor Nabor Nabor
  [1,]      1     8    11     3     6
  [2,]      2     3     9     5     4
  [3,]      3     8     6     9     2
  [4,]      4     5     7     9    10
  [5,]      5     4     9     7    10
  [6,]      6    10     8     3     9
  [7,]      7     4     5    10     9
  [8,]      8    11     6     3    10
  [9,]      9     5    10     4     7
 [10,]     10     7     6     9     5
 [11,]     11     8     6     1     3
```

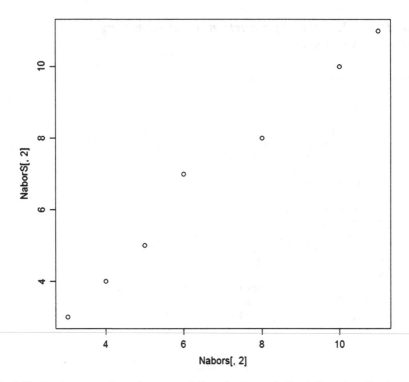

Fig. 5.11 Contingent numbers of nearest neighbors in six standardized dimensions (*horizontal*) versus two principal coordinate dimensions (*vertical*). Some points are multiples

An immediate use for near neighbor analysis is to investigate whether, and if so how, the recasting of contingent centroids from six standardized dimensions into two principal coordinate dimensions has affected the nearest neighbor relations among the contingents. This can be determined by getting neighbors of the six-dimensional structure, and then plotting nearest neighbor contingent numbers against each other as in Fig. 5.11.

```
@ Nabors <- Naboring(Centr11S)
@ plot(Nabors[,2],NaborS[,2])
```

The only perturbation of (first) nearest neighbor relations by principal coordinate dimensional reduction is for contingent number 10, which originally had contingent 6 as nearest neighbor that switched to contingent 7. The original nearest neighbor has become the second nearest neighbor, but contingent 7 was originally not even among the four near neighbors to contingent 10. The PCO process has done more extensive perturbation to higher order neighbor relations as shown for second nearest neighbors in Fig. 5.12. Thus, it is better to compile the k-neighbor data from the full set of variates.

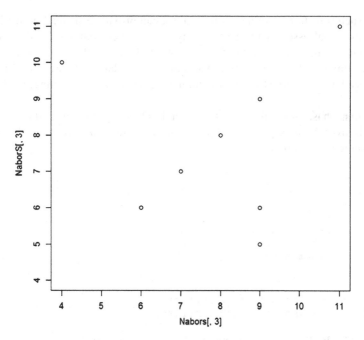

Fig. 5.12 Contingent numbers of second nearest neighbors in six standardized dimensions (*horizontal*) versus two principal coordinate dimensions (*vertical*). Some points are multiples

```
@ Nabors
        Locus Nabor Nabor Nabor Nabor
 [1,]      1     8    11     3     6
 [2,]      2     3     9     5     4
 [3,]      3     8     6     2     9
 [4,]      4     5     7     9    10
 [5,]      5     4     9    10     7
 [6,]      6    10     8     3     9
 [7,]      7     4     9    10     5
 [8,]      8    11     6     3    10
 [9,]      9     5     4    10     7
[10,]     10     6     9     5     4
[11,]     11     8     6     1     3
```

Skeletal Subset as Comparative Core

It would be somewhat unusual to find a dataset in which all contingents were insensitive in this network sense to standardization of the variates. It would also be somewhat unusual to find a dataset without a substantial subset that does not exhibit such sensitivity. An insensitive subset can provide a skeletal network that facilitates visual assessment of sensitivity in the other contingents. For current contingents, a subset consisting of contingents 1, 2, 3, 4, 8, 9, and 11 has the same neighbor linkages for both original variates and standardized variates. This provides a skeletal network structure for comparing sensitivity of contingents 5, 6, 7, and 10.

The first phase of configuring the skeletal network is to extract the subset of centroids from both original and standardized scalings, and then to obtain the NaborNet for each subset.

```
@ #Specity subset.
@ PCOss <- c(1,2,3,4,8,9,11)
@ #Extract subsets of centroids.
@ PCOcntr11ss <- PCOcntr11[PCOss,]
@ PCOcntr11Sss <- PCOcntr11S[PCOss,]
@ #Compute NaborNet for each subset.
@ source("NetWorks.txt")


@ NetFram <- NaborNet(PCOcntr11ss)
@ NetFramS <- NaborNet(PCOcntr11Sss)
@ NetFram
      NetNode NetLink NetOrder  LinkDist Nabor
[1,]        1       5         1 0.8970156     1
[2,]        2       3         5 1.1756613     1
[3,]        3       5         4 1.0788562     1
[4,]        4       6         7 0.8008658     1
[5,]        5       1         2 0.8970156     2
[6,]        6       3         6 1.3419343     2
[7,]        7       5         3 0.8086512     1
@ NetFramS
      NetNode NetLink NetOrder  LinkDist Nabor
[1,]        1       5         1 1.3917978     1
[2,]        2       3         7 1.0237637     1
[3,]        3       5         4 0.8576501     1
[4,]        4       6         6 0.6709109     1
[5,]        5       1         2 1.3917978     3
[6,]        6       3         5 0.9551064     2
[7,]        7       5         3 0.7089732     1
```

The second phase is to superimpose the network linkages for a subset on a plot showing centroids for all of the contingents in that particular scaling. This process is as follows for the original variates, producing Fig. 5.13. Note particularly the need to reference actual contingent numbers rather than sequential numbers in the NetFrame for the subset.

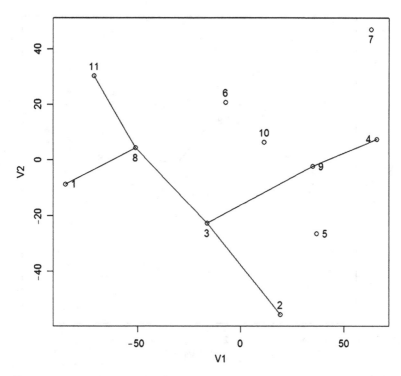

Fig. 5.13 PCO centroids of contingents based on original variates showing skeletal network of consistent contingents

```
@ plot(PCOcntr11)
@ identify(PCOcntr11)
 [1]  1  2  3  4  5  6  7  8  9 10 11
@ Nodess <- length(NetFram[,1])
@ for(I in 1:Nodess)
@@ {J <- NetFram[I,1]
@@ #Get contingent number.
@@   J <- PCOss[J]
@@   K <- NetFram[I,2]
@@ #Get contingent number.
@@   K <- PCOss[K]
@@   X <- c(PCOcntr11[J,1],PCOcntr11[K,1])
@@   Y <- c(PCOcntr11[J,2],PCOcntr11[K,2])
@@   lines(X,Y)
@@ }
```

The corresponding plotting scenario for contingents based on standardized variates is as follows to produce Fig. 5.14:

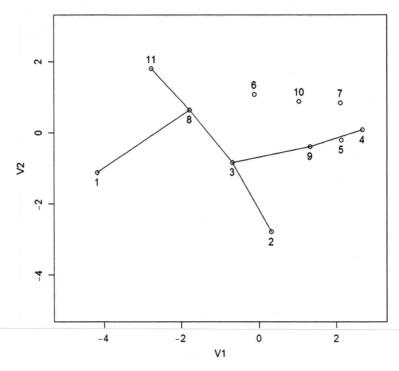

Fig. 5.14 PCO centroids of contingents based on standardized variates showing skeletal network of consistent contingents

```
@ plot(PCOcntr11S,xlim=c(-5,3),ylim=c(-5,3))
@ identify(PCOcntr11S)
 [1]  1  2  3  4  5  6  7  8  9 10 11
@ for(I in 1:Nodess)
@@ {J <- NetFramS[I,1]
@@  J <- PCOss[J]
@@  K <- NetFramS[I,2]
@@  K <- PCOss[K]
@@  X <- c(PCOcntr11S[J,1],PCOcntr11S[K,1])
@@  Y <- c(PCOcntr11S[J,2],PCOcntr11S[K,2])
@@  lines(X,Y)
@@ }
```

Comparing Figs. 5.13 and 5.14 makes clear the nearly linear sequence of links from contingent 2 to contingent 11 through contingents 3 and 8 with a single-step left branch from contingent 8 to contingent 1 and a two-step right branch from contingent 3 to contingent 4 through contingent 9. Contingents 6, 7, and 10 are above the right branch for both scalings, and contingent 5 is below the right branch for both scalings. However, contingent 5 is almost on the right branch for standardized scaling, whereas it is appreciably below for original scaling. Likewise, contingent 7 is almost directly to the right of contingents 6 and 10 for standardized scaling, whereas it is shifted substantially above and to the right for original scaling. Thus, original scaling gives more distinctiveness to contingents 5 and 7 than does standardized scaling.

Sequence Scaling and Representative Ranks

A process of prioritization entails comparing either cases or collectives of cases in terms of the information imbedded in the multiple measures. Collectives of cases form constellations in the space of multiple measures, and centroids constitute cores of those constellations. Centroids are, thus, conceptually compatible for such comparisons. Distance domains abstracted from centroid-to-centroid distances deal directly with the comparative concerns without being tightly tied to the multiple measures, and so are also appropriate for prioritization purposes.

We have empirical evidence that standardized scaling has effects expressed in the distance domains. We have also seen that standardized scalings are completely correlated with original observations. Thus, complete correlation does not carry complete consistency for comparison. A common component of information in original and standardized scales is specification of "greater than," "less than," and "equal to" relationships among the instances, although there are disparate degrees of difference. Rankings retain only object ordering information, and can therefore be considered as a "bare bones" sequence scaling or skeletal scaling.

Rankings can rise with magnitude of measurement which is the regular ranking for **R** or can carry context of precedence in placement with first as foremost and largest as least precedence. Preferential positioning properties make place ranks a better basis for prioritization purposes. Function 5.3 is a PlacRank facility that takes a data frame of variate values as input and produces a data frame of place ranks as outputs.

Function 5.3: PlacRank Function for Converting a Data Frame to Place Ranks

```
PlacRank <- function(Ratings)
{Rated <- length(Ratings)
 Cases <- length(Ratings[,1])
 Ranked <- Ratings
 for(I in 1:Rated)
  Ranked[,I] <- (Cases+1) - rank(Ratings[,I],ties.method="average")
 Ranked
}
```

If place ranks for all variates have the same sense of superiority, they become a kind of common currency for comparative purposes in prioritization. This requires each variate to be considered in a criterion context as an informational indicator. For example, the percent in one forest patch and the percent in one open patch are inherently inverse indicators as evidenced by their strong negative correlation. Comparative coupling of inverse indicators must either be done through a distance domain or the inversions must be inverted. In terms of sequence scaling, regular rankings of inverse indicators are compatible with place rankings of those that have positive polarity.

Since standardization does not do any reordering, mixed-mode rankings (not necessarily same sense) are identical whether obtained from original observations or standardized scales.

```
@ MixModeRnks <- PlacRank(Centr11)
@ MixModeRnks
   BirdSp MamlSp ElevSD PctFor Pct1FPch Pct1OPch
1     11     11     11     10       10        2
2     10      9      8      1        2       10
3      9     10     10      7        7        5
4      4      1      2      2        1       11
5      2      4      6      3        3        9
6      1      6      4      8        8        4
7      5      2      1      5        5        7
8      8      8      9      9        9        3
9      7      5      3      4        4        8
10     3      3      5      6        6        6
11     6      7      7     11       11        1

@ sum(MixModeRnkS - MixModeRnks)
[1] 0
```

Furthermore, it is seen that same-sense rankings of Pct1FPch and Pct1OPch are identical and, therefore, redundant for rank-based prioritization purposes.

```
@ cbind(MixModeRnks[,5],rank(Centr11[,6]))
       [,1] [,2]
 [1,]    10   10
 [2,]     2    2
 [3,]     7    7
 [4,]     1    1
 [5,]     3    3
 [6,]     8    8
 [7,]     5    5
 [8,]     9    9
 [9,]     4    4
[10,]     6    6
[11,]    11   11
```

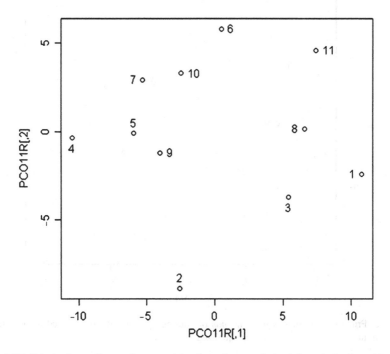

Fig. 5.15 Principal coordinates for centroids of contingents derived from (mixed mode) place ranks

For comparative continuity, a distance domain is also obtained for centroids expressed in terms of ranks as shown in Fig. 5.15.

```
@ Dist11R <- dist(MixModeRnks,method="euclidean")
@ PCO11R <- cmdscale(Dist11R)
@ plot(PCO11R)
@ identify(PCO11R)
```

The plot in Fig. 5.15 shows that the first (horizontal) PCO axis requires reversal, which is done as follows and plotted in Fig. 5.16.

```
@ PCOcntr11R <- as.data.frame(PCO11R)
@ PCOcntr11R[,1] <- -1.0 * PCOcntr11R[,1]
@ plot(PCOcntr11R,ylim=c(-10,10))
@ identify(PCOcntr11R)
```

The skeletal subset used earlier is superimposed in Fig. 5.17. Figure 5.17 is more like the version for standardized data than for original observations, except that contingent 5 is located slightly above the link line instead of slightly below.

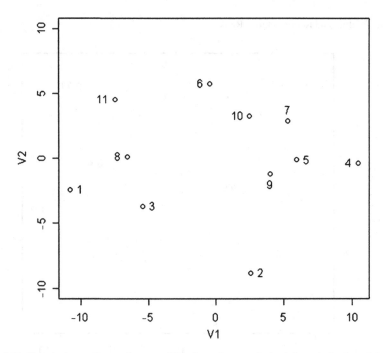

Fig. 5.16 Principal coordinates for centroids of contingents derived from (mixed mode) place ranks with first axis inverted and ranges equalized

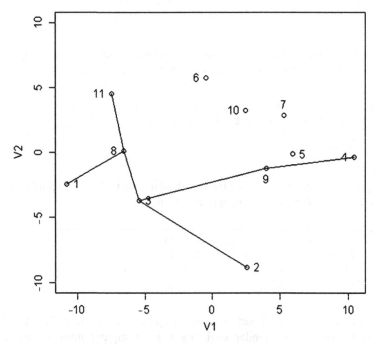

Fig. 5.17 Principal coordinates for centroids of contingents derived from (mixed mode) place ranks with first axis adjustment and showing prior skeletal network

Both standardization and ranking have equilibrating effects on variability, but these effects are different. Since it has already been shown that Pct1FPch and Pct1OPch are rank equivalent at the level of contingents, Pct1OPch should simply be omitted for rank-based comparative purposes. This omission gives same-sense structure to the remaining ranks.

In general, mixed modes for rankings should be resolved by substituting regular rankings for place-based rankings of those individual variates that are counter-indicative. It should also be noted that retaining redundant variates has the effect of more heavily weighting the influences that give rise to the redundancies.

Representative Ranks

Ranks solely signify sequences, thus constituting conceptual common currency for prioritization purposes. Consider **k** contingents of cases, with each case having same-sense ranks on **p** variates. If the **j**th contingent consists of $\mathbf{h}_j$ cases, there are $\mathbf{h}_j \times \mathbf{p} = \mathbf{q}_j$ rank numbers associated with the contingent. If these $\mathbf{q}_j$ rank numbers are placed in a single array and sorted in ascending order, they form a distribution of rank values for the contingent. A selected set of $\mathbf{m} \leq \mathbf{q}_j$ percentage points for this distribution can be considered as representative ranks for the contingent. Then, contingents can be prioritized comparatively in terms of their representative ranks (Myers and Patil 2010; Myers et al. 2006; Sorensen et al. 2005).

To pursue representative ranks, we obtain a data frame of place ranks for cases on the first five variates as follows:

```
@ CasPlacRnk5 <- PlacRank(BAMBI[,2:6])
@ CasPlacRnk5 <- cbind(BAMBI[,1],CasPlacRnk5)
@ names(CasPlacRnk5)[1] <- "HexID"
@ head(CasPlacRnk5)
  HexID BirdSp MamlSp ElevSD PctFor Pct1FPch
1  1714  211.0  210.5  211.0  193.0      170
2  1827  210.0  205.0  190.5   69.0       67
3  1828  159.0  205.0  199.5  165.0      147
4  1829  202.5  210.5  208.0  202.0      187
5  1941  204.0  205.0  134.5    2.0        2
6  1942  148.0  187.0  179.0  106.5       92
```

Function 5.4 is a GroupRnk function that compiles five representative ranks for collectives. The five key ranks are (1) minimum rank, (2) first quartile rank, (3) median rank, (4) third quartile rank, and (5) maximum rank. The inputs to the function are a vector of group membership and a data frame of case-level same-sense ranks of criteria.

Function 5.4: GroupRnk Function for Compiling Key Ranks
of Collectives (Minimum, First Quartile, Median, Third Quartile,
and Maximum) from Case-Level Rankings

```
GroupRnk <- function(Membrshp,CasRnks)
{Groups <- max(Membrshp)
 GroupSiz <- rep(0,Groups)
 Cases <- length(Membrshp)
 Casings <- length(CasRnks)
 for(I in 1:Groups)
  {J <- Membrshp[I]
   GroupSiz[J] <- GroupSiz[J] + 1
  }
 Min <- rep(0,Groups)
 Q1 <- rep(0,Groups)
 Med <- rep(0,Groups)
 Q3 <- rep(0,Groups)
 Max <- rep(0,Groups)
 KeyRnks <- cbind(Min,Q1,Med,Q3,Max)
 for(I in 1:Groups)
  {RnkValus <- GroupSiz[I] * Casings
   RnkList <- rep(0,RnkValus)
   ListIndx <- 0
   for(J in 1:Cases)
    {if(Membrshp[J]==I)
      {for(K in 1:Casings)
        {ListIndx <- ListIndx+1
         RnkList[ListIndx] <- CasRnks[J,K]
        }
      }
    }
   KeyRnks[I,1] <- round(min(RnkList),1)
   KeyRnks[I,2] <- round(quantile(RnkList,probs=0.25),1)
   KeyRnks[I,3] <- round(median(RnkList),1)
   KeyRnks[I,4] <- round(quantile(RnkList,probs=0.75),1)
   KeyRnks[I,5] <- round(max(RnkList),1)
  }
 KeyRnks
}
```

Function 5.4 is applied to the 11 contingents as follows, with pairs plotted in Fig. 5.18.

Figure 5.18 shows that plotting Q3 on the vertical against the median on the horizontal yields a near-linear ordering of the contingents. The plot is extracted and labeled in Fig. 5.19.

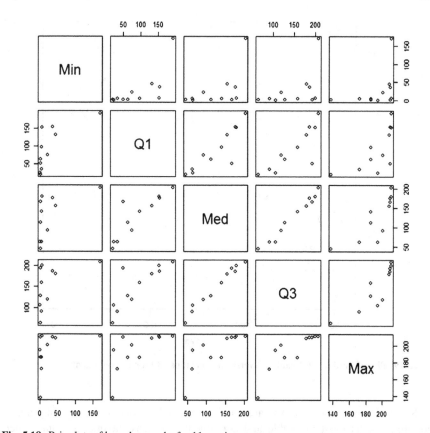

Fig. 5.18 Pair plots of key place ranks for 11 contingents

```
@ source("NearNabr.txt")
@ NaborS <- Naboring(PCOcntr11S)
@ NaborS
      Locus Nabor Nabor Nabor Nabor
 [1,]     1     8    11     3     6
 [2,]     2     3     9     5     4
 [3,]     3     8     6     9     2
 [4,]     4     5     7     9    10
 [5,]   4.0  34.5  62.0  91.0 172.0
 [6,]   4.5  97.0 140.0 158.5 185.5
 [7,]   1.0  24.5  63.0 106.0 194.5
 [8,]  36.0 155.0 175.5 186.5 210.0
 [9,]  21.5  75.4  91.5 119.0 201.0
[10,]   1.5  62.8 112.0 128.1 185.5
[11,]   6.5 152.5 179.0 200.0 211.0
@ pairs(KeyRnks11)
```

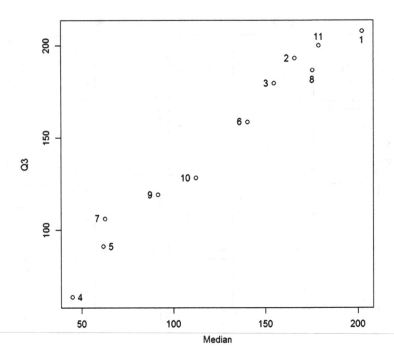

Fig. 5.19 Plot of third quartile rank (Y) versus median rank (X) for 11 contingents

Since lower place ranks are more favorable, this ordering highlights contingent 4 as most favorable and contingent 1 as least favorable. Some other pairings of key ranks make the contingents appear less distinctive.

References

Borg I, Groenen P (2005) Modern multidimensional scaling: theory and applications, 2nd edn. Springer-Verlag, New York

Cox T, Cox M (2001) Multidimensional scaling. Chapman & Hall/CRC, Boca Raton, FL

Green P, Carmone F, Smith S (1989) Multidimensional scaling: concepts and applications. Allyn & Bacon, Boston, MA

Myers W, Patil GP (2010) Preliminary prioritization based on partial order theory and **R** software for compositional complexes in landscape ecology, with applications to restoration, remediation, and enhancement. Environ Ecol Stat 17:411–436

Myers W, Patil GP, Cai Y (2006) Exploring patterns of habitat diversity across landscapes using partial ordering. In: Brüggemann R, Carlsen L (eds) Partial order in environmental sciences and chemistry. Springer, Berlin, pp 309–325

Sorensen P, Brüggemann RM, Thomsen LD (2005) Applications of multidimensional rank-correlation. Match Commun Math Comput Chem 54(3):643–670

Wu B, Chao K-M (2004) Spanning trees and optimization problems. CRC Press, Boca Raton, FL

Zuur A, Ieno E, Smith G (2007) Analyzing ecological data. Springer, New York

Part II
Precedence and Progressive Prioritization

Chapter 6
Ascribed Advantage, Subordination Schematic, and ORDIT Ordering

The foregoing treatments have set the stage for a more formal approach to precedence and partial/progressive prioritization that has its foundation in partial order analysis (Brüggemann and Voigt 2008; Brüggemann and Patil 2011; De Loof et al. 2008; Patil and Taillie 2004). We wish to formalize favorability without specifying exactly how it is to be determined, leaving latitude for investigative innovation and interpretation. Our approach here is comparative among contingents or cases, and is framed in terms of *ascribed advantage* that is an outcome of a *rating regime* (Myers and Patil 2010).

Ascribed Advantage, Subordinate Status, and Indefinite Instances

We assume the availability of a suite of rating rules that assigns three types of relations between a particular pair of cases or contingents (instances), with the two members of the pair being symbolized as Э and Є. If the rules designate Э as more favorable than Є, then we say that Э is/has *ascribed advantage* over Є which we symbolize as:

ЭaaЄ, wherein Э is *ascribed advantage* over Є

which also implies that Є has *subordinate status* relative to Э symbolized as:

ЄssЭ, wherein Є has *subordinate status* to Э which reciprocally implies ЭaaЄ.

In simple terms, ascribed advantage means more favorable and subordinate status means less favorable according to the regime of rating rules. However, the rating rules may fail to ascribe advantage and subordinate status for a particular pair of instances. These latter are *indefinite instances* symbolized as:

ЭiiЄ, whereby these are *indefinite instances* without ascribed advantage and without subordinate status, which reciprocally implies ЄiiЭ.

W.L. Myers and G.P. Patil, *Multivariate Methods of Representing Relations in R for Prioritization Purposes*, Environmental and Ecological Statistics 6, DOI 10.1007/978-1-4614-3122-0_6, © Springer Science+Business Media, LLC 2012

Indefinite instances are pairs for which the rating rules fail to assign advantage.

Each of the **n** cases or contingents can be compared on this basis to all others in the deleted domain **DD** = **n** − 1 of competing cases (instances) with the percent occurrence of these relations being tabulated as follows, where $ff(\ )$ denotes focal frequency as number of occurrences for the focal case:

$$\mathbf{AA} = 100 \times ff(\text{aa}) / \mathbf{DD}.$$

$$\mathbf{SS} = 100 \times ff(\text{ss}) / \mathbf{DD}.$$

$$\mathbf{II} = 100 \times ff(\text{ii}) / \mathbf{DD}.$$

Clearly, **AA** + **SS** + **II** = 100%; and for later use, let us define **CCC** = 100 − **AA** as the *complement of case condition relative to ascribed advantage* (**AA**).

In the parlance of partial order, AA has sense of relative size of deleted "down set," SS has sense of relative size of deleted "up set," and II has parallels to cases with conflicting criteria. Since AA, SS, and II can be computed individually for any instance, this approach is in the nature of a local partial order model (LPOM).

Subordination Schematic

The foregoing approach can be symbolized schematically in what we call a "subordination schematic" as depicted in Fig. 6.1, whereby the point representing an instance partitions the figure into a "trapezoidal triplet" (of AA, SS, and II) below, and a "topping triangle" (of CCC, SS, and II) above. The combination of lower and

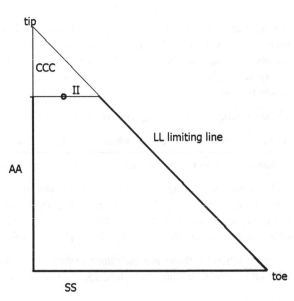

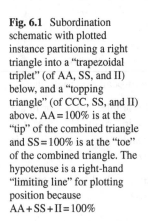

Fig. 6.1 Subordination schematic with plotted instance partitioning a right triangle into a "trapezoidal triplet" (of AA, SS, and II) below, and a "topping triangle" (of CCC, SS, and II) above. AA = 100% is at the "tip" of the combined triangle and SS = 100% is at the "toe" of the combined triangle. The hypotenuse is a right-hand "limiting line" for plotting position because AA + SS + II = 100%

upper portions forms a right triangle with the "tip" at AA = 100% in the upper left and the "toe" at SS = 100% in the lower right. The hypotenuse is a right-hand "limiting line" for plotting position because AA + SS + II = 100%. CCC adds SS + II to AA making 100%. The "basal bar" (bottom leg) of the topping triangle is partitioned into SS and II by the plotted point for the instance.

The trapezoidal triplet is used subsequently as the basis for a precedence plot. The topping triangle provides the basis for an "Ordering Dually in Triangles, ORDIT, ordering" of the instances as explained immediately below.

Ordering Dually in Triangles

For the current context, an ideal instance is taken to be one that has ascribed advantage over all others. In terms of rating relations as set forth above, this is an instance for which AA is 100% of the deleted domain (DD) of other instances, that is, the frequency of ascribed advantage being equal to the number of competing cases (instances). When this ideal actually occurs, then the trapezoidal triplet becomes a triangle. Whether or not the ideal actually occurs, this can be cast in terms of a "topping triangle" for each instance that puts a triangular vertex in place when overlaid on the trapezoid as shown in Fig. 6.1.

The legs of the topping triangle can be coupled as a decimal value **ccc.bbb** for each part of which lower values are more favorable in company with place-based rankings. The **ccc** component is obtained by rounding CCC to two decimal places and then multiplying by 100. The **bbb** component is obtained by dividing SS by CCC, and imposing 0.999 as an upper limit. The two components are then coupled by adding **bbb** to **ccc**. Each instance induces a topping triangle, so this ordering is assigned the acronym **ORDIT** for ORdering Dually In Triangles. It preserves all aspects of AA, SS, and II, except for the actual number of instances. If a simple sequencing of instances is needed, then the ORDITs can be converted to regular ranks. Regular ranking of the ORDITs is done because the polarity of ORDITs is to be preserved.

Product-Order Rating Regime

A general relational rule for ascribing advantage is *product order*, whereby advantage is gained by having all criteria at least as good and at least one better. Conversely, subordinate status lies with having all criteria at least as poor and at least one poorer. This relational rule is applicable to all kinds of criteria as long as they have the same polarity (same sense of better and worse). We have chosen to refer to regular ranks of ORDITs based on product order as *salient scaling*. Function 6.1 is a ProdOrdr facility that determines ORDITs and salient scaling according to product order.

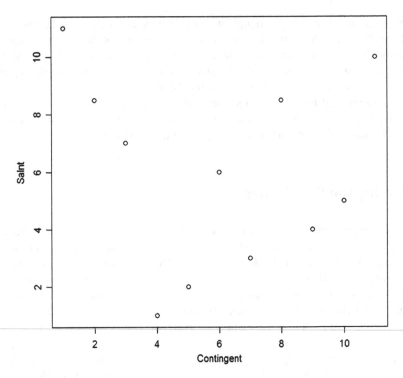

Fig. 6.2 Salient scaling (prioritization) for contingents based on representative (place based) ranks Q2 (median) and Q3

This function takes as its inputs a vector of IDs for instances, a data frame of same-sense criteria, and an indicator of whether the criteria are positive sense (placing $=0$) or negative sense (placing $=1$). The output is a data frame of ORDITs and salient scaling values.

We concluded the previous chapter by examining a plot of (place based) third-quartile ranks versus median ranks for contingents which showed a near-linear relationship suggesting that these two criteria serve to produce a precedence ordering that distinguishes among the contingents. We use this as an initial exploration of prioritization at the contingent level shown in Fig. 6.2.

```
@ source("ProdOrdr.txt")
@ PlacBased <- 1
@ Salnt11Q2Q3 <- ProdOrdr(CntngnID,KeyRnks11[,3:4],PlacBased)
@ plot(Salnt11Q2Q3[,5],xlab="Contingent",ylab="Salnt")
```

Function 6.1: ProdOrdr Function for ORDIT Ordering and Salient Scaling According to Product-Order Protocols

```
ProdOrdr <- function(CaseIDs,Ratings,Placing)
{Ncol <- length(Ratings)
 Ncase <- length(Ratings[,1])
 Status1 <- rep(-1,Ncase)
 Status2 <- Status1
 DD <- Ncase - 1
 for(I in 1:Ncase)
  {Nosub <- 0; Levl <- 0
   for(J in 1:Ncase)
    {if(I<J | I>J)
      {MatchA <- 0; MatchB <- 0; Undom <- 1
       VecA <- Ratings[I,] - Ratings[J,]
       if(Placing>0) VecA <- Ratings[J,] - Ratings[I,]
       if(max(VecA) > 0) MatchA <- 1
       if(min(VecA) < 0) MatchB <- 1
       if(MatchA==1 & MatchB==0) Nosub <- Nosub + 1
       if(MatchA==0 & MatchB==1) Undom <- 0
       Levl <- Levl + Undom
      }
    }
   Status1[I] <- Nosub
   Status2[I] <- DD - Levl
  }
 AA <- Status1
 SS <- Status2
 Pct <- 100/DD
 AA <- AA * Pct
 AA <- round(AA,digits=2)
 SS <- SS * Pct
 SS <- round(SS,digits=2)
 ccc <- rep(0,Ncase)
 bbb <- ccc
 ORDIT <- ccc
 for(I in 1:Ncase)
  {ccc[I] <- (100 - AA[I]) * 100
   ccc[I] <- round(ccc[I],digits=0)
   if(AA[I] < 100) bbb[I] <- SS[I]/(100 - AA[I])
   if(bbb[I] > 0.999) bbb[I] <- 0.999
   bbb[I] <- round(bbb[I],digits=3)
   ORDIT[I] <- ccc[I] + bbb[I]
  }
 Salnt <- rank(ORDIT)
 Salients <- cbind(CaseIDs,AA,SS,ORDIT,Salnt)
 Salients
}
```

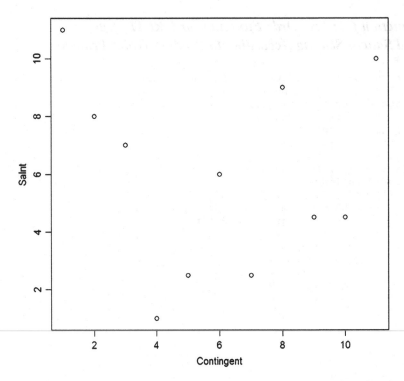

Fig. 6.3 Salient scaling (prioritization) for contingents based on representative (place based) ranks Q1, Q2 (median), and Q3

One proceeds interpretively from bottom to top in Fig. 6.2. Contingents 4, 5, and 7 are first, second, and third, respectively, according to Q2 and Q3 with the only lack of resolution being between contingents 2 and 8. If Q1 is included in the prioritization, the result becomes as shown in Fig. 6.3.

```
@ Salnt11Q1Q2Q3 <- ProdOrdr(CntngnID,KeyRnks11[,2:4],PlacBased)
@ plot(Salnt11Q1Q2Q3[,5],xlab="Contingent",ylab="Salnt")
```

Including Q1 resolves contingents 2 and 8 by placing 2 before 8, but induces confounding of contingent 5 with contingents 7 and 9 with contingent 10. Contingent 4 still stands alone as first.

The three varieties of principal coordinate distance domains can be investigated comparatively in this regard if it is remembered that the polarity of the PCOs is opposite that of place ranks. A pairs plot is given in Fig. 6.4.

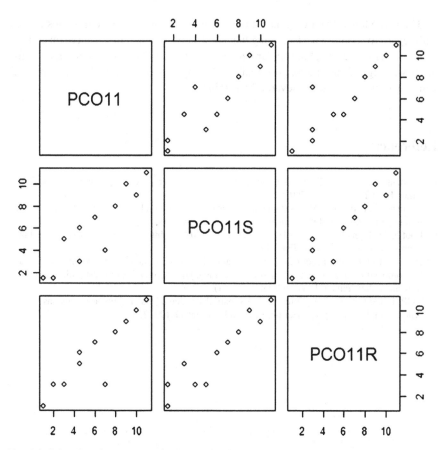

Fig. 6.4 Pairs plot of prioritizations of contingents from PCO distance domains

```
@ PlacBasd <- 0
@ SalntPCO11 <- ProdOrdr(CntngnID,PCOcntr11,PlacBasd)
@ SalntPCO11S <- ProdOrdr(CntngnID,PCOcntr11S,PlacBasd)
@ SalntPCO11R <- ProdOrdr(CntngnID,PCOcntr11R,PlacBasd)
@ SalntPCO <- cbind(SalntPCO11[,5],SalntPCO11S[,5],SalntPCO11R[,5])
@ SalntPCO <- as.data.frame(SalntPCO)
@ names(SalntPCO) <- cbind("PCO11","PCO11S","PCO11R")
@ SalntPCO
   PCO11 PCO11S PCO11R
1   11.0   11.0     11
2    9.0   10.0      9
3   10.0    9.0     10
4    2.0    1.5      3
5    7.0    4.0      3
6    3.0    5.0      3
7    1.0    1.5      1
8    8.0    8.0      8
9    4.5    6.0      6
10   4.5    3.0      5
11   6.0    7.0      7
@ pairs(SalntPCO)
```

The precedence from original, standardized, and rank distance domains agrees with regard to (contingent 1 as being the worst). Original and ranks agree on contingent 7 as being the best, but standardized has contingent 7 tied with contingent 4 for the best. Original and ranks are in substantial agreement, except for contingent 5 which is third by ranks but seventh by original.

References

Brüggemann R, Voigt K (2008) Basic principles of Hasse diagram technique in chemistry. Comb Chem High T Scr 11:756–769

Brüggemann R, Patil GP (2011) Ranking and prioritization with multi-indicator systems, introduction to partial order and its applications. Springer, New York

De Loof K, De Baets B, De Meyer H, Brüggemann R (2008) A hitchhiker's guide to poset ranking. Comb Chem High T Scr 11:734–744

Myers W, Patil GP (2010) Preliminary prioritization based on partial order theory and R software for compositional complexes in landscape ecology, with applications to restoration, remediation, and enhancement. Environ Ecol Stat 17(4)

Patil GP, Taillie C (2004) Multiple indicators, partially ordered sets, and linear extensions: multi-criterion ranking and prioritization. Environ Ecol Stat 11:199–228

Chapter 7
Precedence Plots, Coordinated Criteria, and Rank Relations

Visualization is an important part of conveying the logic of a prioritization to constituent stakeholders (Brüggemann and Patil 2010; Brüggemann et al. 2003). Therefore, we exploit the concept of trapezoidal triplet (see Fig. 6.1) to prepare an innovative precedence plot before going forward with comparison of contingents in terms of ORDITs under alternative rating regimes (Myers and Patil 2010).

Precedence Plots

Function 7.1 named TrpzTrpl (for trapezoidal triplet) accepts the output of the ProdOrdr function (6.1) and produces a precedence plot. This is applied to second- and third-quartile representative ranks and shown in Fig. 7.1.

Function 7.1: TrpzTrpl Function for Precedence Plots Based on Trapezoidal Triplet

```
TrpzTrpl <- function(AaSs)
# Input is data frame of rating relations.
# Idz is column number of CaseIDs.
# Aa is column number of AA.
# Ss is column number of SS.
{Cases <- length(AaSs[,1])
 Idz <- 1
 Aa <- 2
 Ss <- 3
 Ymax <- max(AaSs[,Aa])
 Ymin <- min(AaSs[,Aa])
```

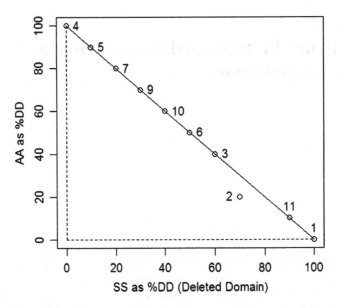

Fig. 7.1 Precedence plot of trapezoidal triplet for contingents based on Q2 and Q3 of representative ranks. *Y*-axis as vertical side is ascribed advantage (AA) as percent of deleted domain (DD) of competing cases. *X*-axis along lower side is subordinate status (SS) as percent of DD. Slanting side is limiting line (LL) for positional plotting. Horizontal distance to limiting line from plotted point (as for contingent 2) may be considered as a "grey gap" due to indefinite instances (II)

```
Xmax <- max(AaSs[,Ss])
Xmin <- min(AaSs[,Ss])
Xright <- Ymax
if(Xmax>Ymax) Xright <- Xmax
plot(AaSs[,Ss],AaSs[,Aa],ylab="AA as %DD",
xlab="SS as %DD (Deleted Domain)",xlim=c(0,Xright))
YY <- c(Ymax,Ymin)
XX <- c(100-Ymax,100-Ymin)
lines(XX,YY,lty=1)
XX <- c(Xmin,Xmin)
YY <- c(Ymin,Ymax)
lines(XX,YY,lty=2)
XX <- c(Xmin,Ymax)
if(Xmax>Ymax) XX <- c(Xmin,Xmax)
YY <- c(Ymin,Ymin)
lines(XX,YY,lty=2)
XX <- c(Xmin,100-Ymax)
YY <- c(Ymax,Ymax)
lines(XX,YY,lty=2)
}
@ TrpzTrpl(Salnt11Q2Q3)
@ identify(Salnt11Q2Q3[,3],Salnt11Q2Q3[,2])
```

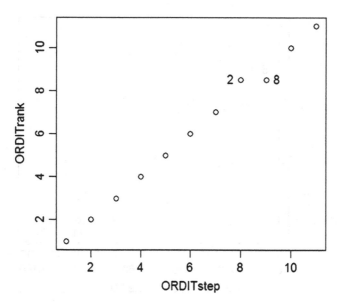

Fig. 7.2 Progression plot for contingents based on Q2 and Q3 of representative ranks with tied contingents identified. Ties occur, where there are two or more successive ORDIT ranks on the same level

Preferential positioning declines downward diagonally from tip to toe. Primary preference varies vertically showing that there is a larger percentage of ascribed advantage with increasing height. *Horizontal variation on a given level shows clarity of comparison. Closer to the limiting line is <u>more definite disadvantage</u>* with a larger percentage of subordinate status versus indefinite instances among the couplets, where ascribed advantage is *lacking. Horizontal distance from limiting line is a "grey gap"* (not black and white) reflecting lack of clarity due to indefinite instances (II) of couplets having conflicts among the criteria.

Only contingent 2 of those identified in the precedence plot of Fig. 7.1 shows a "grey gap" of uncertainty due to indefinite instances (II). However, contingent 8 is not identified in Fig. 7.1, so it must be tied with another contingent. In the previous chapter, it was determined that the tie is with contingent 2.

It is expedient to have a companion "progression plot" (progressing from best to worst) for the precedence plot that reveals the presence of ties. A progression plot is obtained by four lines of **R** code as follows and shown in Fig. 7.2.

```
@ ORDITrank <- rank(Salnt11Q2Q3[,4])
@ ORDITstep <- rank(Salnt11Q2Q3[,4],ties.method="first")
@ plot(ORDITstep,ORDITrank)
@ identify(ORDITstep,ORDITrank)
```

Including Q1 with Q2 and Q3 gives the precedence plot shown in Fig. 7.3 and the companion progression plot in Fig. 7.4. This inclusion leaves only contingents

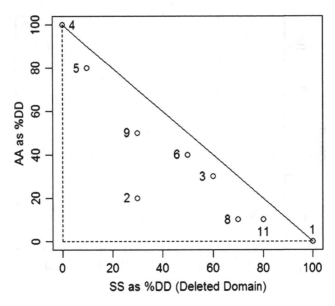

Fig. 7.3 Precedence plot of trapezoidal triplet for contingents based on Q1, Q2, and Q3 of representative ranks

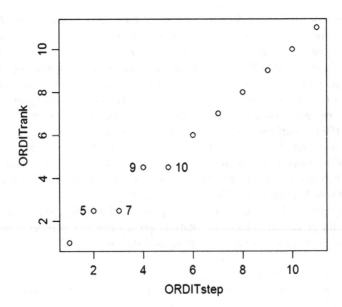

Fig. 7.4 Progression plot for contingents based on Q1, Q2, and Q3 of representative ranks with tied contingents identified

4 and 1 as being without indefinite instances, and contingents 7 and 10 being masked by coincidence (7 with 5 and 10 with 9).

The quartiles of representative ranks, thus, give clear preference to contingent 4 followed dually by contingents 5 and 7. This perspective has contingent 1 in the poorest position.

```
@ TrpzTrpl(Salnt11Q1Q2Q3)
@ identify(Salnt11Q1Q2Q3[,3],Salnt11Q1Q2Q3[,2])

@ ORDITrank <- rank(Salnt11Q1Q2Q3[,4])
@ ORDITstep <- rank(Salnt11Q1Q2Q3[,4],ties.method="first")
@ plot(ORDITstep,ORDITrank)
@ identify(ORDITstep,ORDITrank)
```

Indicator Integration and Condensation

We next undertake integration and condensation (Luther et al. 2000) of principal coordinates across the three distance domains. This begins with constructing a conjunctive data frame as follows, after which the (Pearson) correlations and (Spearman) rank correlations are explored.

```
@ PCOcombo <- cbind(PCOcntr11,PCOcntr11S,PCOcntr11R)
@ names(PCOcombo) <- cbind("PCO11a","PCO11b","PCO11Sa","PCO11Sb",
@@ "PCO11Ra","PCO11Rb")
@ names(PCOcombo)
[1] "PCO11a"  "PCO11b"  "PCO11Sa" "PCO11Sb" "PCO11Ra" "PCO11Rb"

@ head(PCOcombo)
        PCO11a      PCO11b    PCO11Sa     PCO11Sb      PCO11Ra     PCO11Rb
1 -85.258738  -8.731896 -4.1958177 -1.11539315 -10.7916053 -2.4230787
2  19.021173 -55.706080  0.3177547 -2.78903408   2.5824030 -8.8566785
3 -16.144474 -22.847221 -0.6917770 -0.83450113  -5.4324821 -3.6998849
4  66.112967   7.428837  2.6746710  0.07931048  10.4522824 -0.3585404
5  36.580981 -26.615366  2.1239898 -0.20235420   5.9283486 -0.1027161
6  -7.300127  20.791998 -0.1220914  1.08294311  -0.4616488  5.7594142

@ round(cor(PCOcombo,method="pearson"),digits=4)
          PCO11a  PCO11b PCO11Sa PCO11Sb PCO11Ra PCO11Rb
PCO11a    1.0000  0.0000  0.9809 -0.1027  0.9669 -0.0587
PCO11b    0.0000  1.0000  0.0101  0.8715 -0.0080  0.8613
PCO11Sa   0.9809  0.0101  1.0000  0.0000  0.9694  0.0333
PCO11Sb  -0.1027  0.8715  0.0000  1.0000 -0.0498  0.9595
PCO11Ra   0.9669 -0.0080  0.9694 -0.0498  1.0000  0.0000
PCO11Rb  -0.0587  0.8613  0.0333  0.9595  0.0000  1.0000

@ round(cor(PCOcombo,method="spearman"),digits=4)
          PCO11a  PCO11b PCO11Sa PCO11Sb PCO11Ra PCO11Rb
PCO11a    1.0000  0.0727  0.9818 -0.0455  0.9909 -0.0636
PCO11b    0.0727  1.0000  0.0455  0.8455 -0.0091  0.7909
PCO11Sa   0.9818  0.0455  1.0000  0.0000  0.9909 -0.0091
PCO11Sb  -0.0455  0.8455  0.0000  1.0000 -0.0727  0.9727
PCO11Ra   0.9909 -0.0091  0.9909 -0.0727  1.0000 -0.0818
PCO11Rb  -0.0636  0.7909 -0.0091  0.9727 -0.0818  1.0000
```

Within each set, the first PCO axis is uncorrelated with the second axis. Between sets, the first PCO axes are very strongly correlated and the second axes are strongly correlated.

We next seek to induce an approximately block diagonal structure for the correlation matrices by rearranging the indicator variates so that the very strongly correlated first PCO axes come first and then the strongly correlated second PCO axes (Mucha 2002).

```
@ PCOblock <- cbind(PCOcntr11[,1],PCOcntr11S[,1],PCOcntr11R[,1],
@@ PCOcntr11[,2],PCOcntr11S[,2],PCOcntr11R[,2])
@ PCOblock <- as.data.frame(PCOblock)
@ names(PCOblock) <- cbind("PCO11a","PCO11Sa","PCO11Ra",
@@ "PCO11b","PCO11Sb","PCO11Rb")
@ round(cor(PCOblock),digits=4)
          PCO11a PCO11Sa PCO11Ra   PCO11b PCO11Sb PCO11Rb
PCO11a    1.0000  0.9809  0.9669   0.0000 -0.1027 -0.0587
PCO11Sa   0.9809  1.0000  0.9694   0.0101  0.0000  0.0333
PCO11Ra   0.9669  0.9694  1.0000  -0.0080 -0.0498  0.0000
PCO11b    0.0000  0.0101 -0.0080   1.0000  0.8715  0.8613
PCO11Sb  -0.1027  0.0000 -0.0498   0.8715  1.0000  0.9595
PCO11Rb  -0.0587  0.0333  0.0000   0.8613  0.9595  1.0000
```

A pairs plot for the blocked PCOs is given in Fig. 7.5.

```
@ pairs(PCOblock)
```

The strong correlations within blocks and the lack of correlation between blocks make it sensible to condense this indicator information via two sets of ORDITs. The three PCO first-axis indicators contribute one ORDIT ordering, and the three PCO second-axis indicators contribute a second ORDIT ordering. These two ORDIT orderings provide an indicator condensation from six to two. The two ORDIT orderings are obtained as follows and plotted in Fig. 7.6.

```
@ PlacBasd <- 0
@ PCOord1 <- ProdOrdr(CntngnID,PCOblock[,1:3],PlacBasd)
@ PCOord2 <- ProdOrdr(CntngnID,PCOblock[,4:6],PlacBasd)
@ plot(PCOord1[,4],PCOord2[,4])
@ identify(PCOord1[,4],PCOord2[,4])
```

As shown in Fig. 7.7, ORDIT ordering from first PCO axes is consistent with that from quartiles of representative ranks with respect to the three best (4, 5, 7) and the three worst (1, 11, 8); however, Fig. 7.6 shows less consistency with regard to ORDIT ordering from second PCO axes. Contingent 7 is moderately well placed for second PCO axes, but contingent 4 is mediocre and contingent 5 is poorly placed. Thus, contingent 4 and contingent 7 appear to be the better candidates for comparisons at the case level.

ORDIT ordering can, thus, serve to coordinate a set of related indicators, thereby providing a single indicator that draws evidence from all members of the parent set. Such integrated indicators can serve as second-order semi-surrogates for the larger

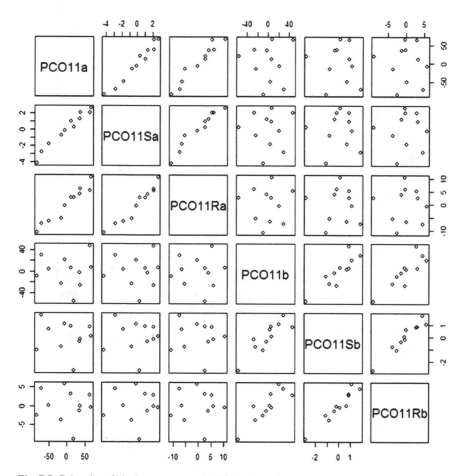

Fig. 7.5 Pairs plot of block arrangement for PCOs of contingents

set of original indicators, whereby implicit weighting due to high redundancies among original indicators has been substantially removed. In the current context, Q1Q2Q3 ORDIT, PCOaxis1 ORDIT, and PCOaxis2 ORDIT can be three second-order indicators for the original nine indicators. This is accomplished as follows, with a precedence plot shown in Fig. 7.8 and companion progression plot in Fig. 7.9. Contingents 7 and 4 appear in positions of precedence.

```
@ CntngOrdr2 <- cbind(Salnt11Q1Q2Q3[,4],PCOord1[,4],PCOord2[,4])
@ CntngOrdr2 <- as.data.frame(CntngOrdr2)
@ names(CntngOrdr2) <- cbind("Q1Q2Q3","PCOaxis1","PCOaxis2")
@ CntngOrdr2
       Q1Q2Q3    PCOaxis1   PCOaxis2
1  10000.999  10000.999   9000.778
2   8000.375   5000.800  10000.999
```

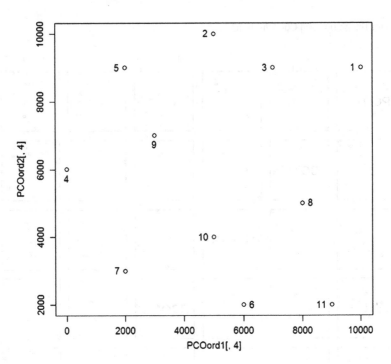

Fig. 7.6 ORDIT ordering from PCO axis 2 (*vertical*) versus ORDIT ordering from PCO axis 1 (*horizontal*)

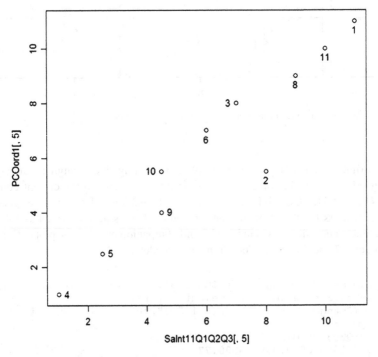

Fig. 7.7 ORDIT rankings from first PCO axis (*Y*) versus ORDIT rankings from quartiles of representative ranks (*X*)

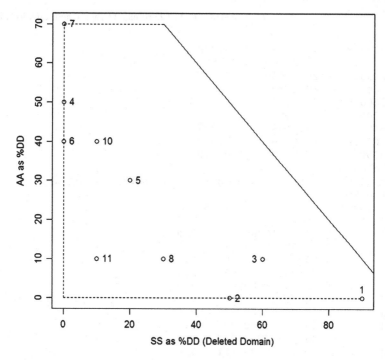

Fig. 7.8 Precedence plot for contingents based on ORDITs as second-order indicators (Q1Q2Q3, PCOaxis1, PCOaxis2)

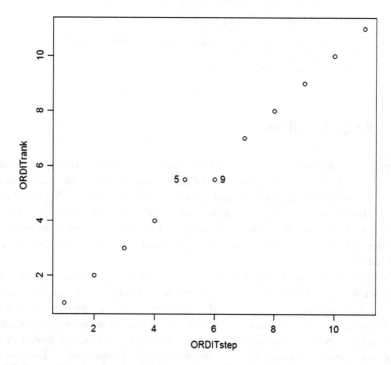

Fig. 7.9 Progression plot showing ties for contingents based on ORDITs as second-order indicators (Q1Q2Q3, PCOaxis1, PCOaxis2)

```
3    7000.857   7000.999   9000.778
4       0.000      0.000   6000.500
5    2000.500   2000.500   9000.556
6    6000.833   6000.999   2000.000
7    2000.500   2000.500   3000.000
8    9000.778   8000.999   5000.800
9    5000.600   3000.999   7000.857
10   5000.600   5000.800   4000.500
11   9000.889   9000.999   2000.000
@ PlacBased <- 1
@ CntngORD2 <- ProdOrdr(CntngnID,CntngOrdr2,PlacBased)
@ CntngORD2
        CaseIDs AA SS      ORDIT Salnt
  [1,]        1  0 90 10000.900   11.0
  [2,]        2  0 50 10000.500   10.0
  [3,]        3 10 60  9000.667    9.0
  [4,]        4 50  0  5000.000    2.0
  [5,]        5 30 20  7000.286    5.5
  [6,]        6 40  0  6000.000    3.0
  [7,]        7 70  0  3000.000    1.0
  [8,]        8 10 30  9000.333    8.0
  [9,]        9 30 20  7000.286    5.5
 [10,]       10 40 10  6000.167    4.0
 [11,]       11 10 10  9000.111    7.0
```

```
@ TrpzTrpl(CntngORD2)
@ identify(CntngORD2[,3],CntngORD2[,2])
 [1]  1  2  3  4  5  6  7  8 10 11
@ ORDITrank <- rank(CntngORD2[,4])
@ ORDITstep <- rank(CntngORD2[,4],ties.method="first")
@ plot(ORDITstep,ORDITrank)
@ identify(ORDITstep,ORDITrank)
```

Rank Range Relations

The product-order rating regime has an alternate interpretation when the indicator criteria consist of a pair of representative ranks, and this alternate interpretation gives rise to a special visualization using what we call "rank rods." One member of a pair of representative ranks is an upper rank, and the other a lower rank. We use the place rank view in what follows, whereby the lower (lesser) rank is the preferred placement and the upper rank is the poorer placement (Newlin et al. 2010; Newlin and Patil 2010).

The rank range is the (closed) interval between the lower and upper ranks or the difference between the maximum and minimum ranks, depending on the context. One instance can be considered better than another in either of the two ways for the rank range sense, depending upon equalities or lack thereof in upper or lower ranks. One instance is better than another in this regard if the lower rank is lower while the upper rank is equal or lower. There is also betterment if upper rank is lower while

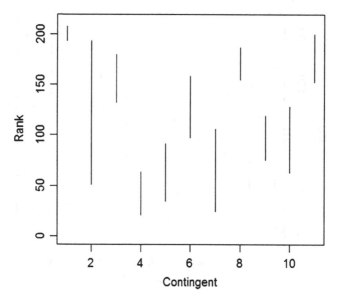

Fig. 7.10 Plot of rank range rods for representative ranks Q1 and Q3

the lower rank is equal or lower. For a pair of representative ranks, application of the rank range rating regime gives equivalent results to product-order regime, and is therefore simply an alternative interpretation.

For the visualization, we proceed to plot a vertical line (rod) for each instance that extends from the level of the lower rank to the level of the upper rank. Q1 and Q3 of the representative ranks for contingents can serve to exemplify this approach according to the following **R** operations with the result shown in Fig. 7.10.

```
@ plot(KeyRnks11[,2],ylim=c(0,211),ylab="Rank",
@@ xlab="Contingent",pch=" ")
@ for(I in 1:11)
@@ {X <- c(I,I)
@@  Y <- c(KeyRnks11[I,2],KeyRnks11[I,4])
@@  lines(X,Y)
@@ }
```

It is evident in Fig. 7.10 that contingent 4 has rank range superiority in terms of representative ranks Q1 and Q3. The nature of the confounding between contingent 5 and contingent 7 for second place is also evident. Contingent 7 is better placed for Q1, but contingent 5 is better placed for Q3. Geometrically, the rank range for contingent 5 is contained within the rank range for contingent 7. Contingent 1 is clearly the worst in both respects. The horizontal axis of Fig. 7.10 is that of an "index plot" in **R**, whereby the numbers simply show the order of occurrence in row of the data.

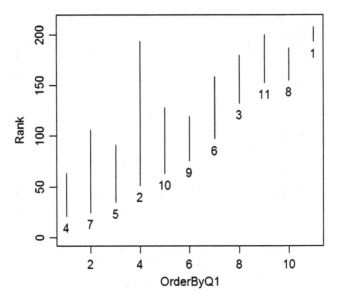

Fig. 7.11 Rank range rods for representative ranks Q1 and Q3 ordered by Q1

It may be desired to have the rank rods ordered otherwise than simple row sequence, as for example by Q1. This can be accomplished as follows and shown in Fig. 7.11.

```
@ OrderByQ1 <- rank(KeyRnks11[,2],ties.method="first")
@ plot(OrderByQ1,KeyRnks11[,2],ylim=c(0,211),ylab="Rank",pch=" ")
@ for(I in 1:11)
@@ {X <- c(OrderByQ1[I],OrderByQ1[I])
@@  Y <- c(KeyRnks11[I,2],KeyRnks11[I,4])
@@   lines(X,Y)
@@ }
@ identify(OrderByQ1,KeyRnks11[,2])
```

With ordering as in Fig. 7.11, a drop in top height for a successor represents confounding, whereby the lower rank and the upper rank present conflicting evidence. A *rank range run* is a sequence of instances, wherein each instance has rank range advantage over its successor in the sequence. Contingent 2 is clearly an anomaly relative to rank range runs, and so would be excluded. A primary rank range run would naturally begin with contingent 4 since it has rank range advantage over all others. Either contingent 7 or contingent 5 would occupy second place since they both have rank range advantage over all remaining, but one or the other would be excluded since they are in conflict. Similarly, either contingent 9 or contingent 10 could be in third place, but they could not both be in the run. Contingent 6 and contingent 3 are then in fourth and fifth place, respectively. Either contingent 11 or contingent 8 could be in sixth place, but they could not both be in the same run. Contingent 1 then occupies the seventh place to terminate the run. The run structure is, thus, 4, (7 or 5), (9 or 10), 6, 3, (11 or 8), 1. Contingent 2 remains an anomaly because of its large span. When ordered by lower rank as in Fig. 7.11, the potential

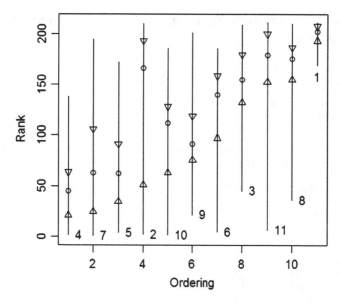

Fig. 7.12 Augmented rank range rods for contingents ordered by Q1. *Rod* extends from minimum rank to maximum rank. *Upward pointing triangle* shows Q1 for ranks. *Downward pointing triangle* shows Q3 for ranks. *Circle* shows median of ranks

successors for an instance in a run can be seen by projecting a horizontal line from the top level. Only those that are transected by the line or entirely above it can serve as successors in a run.

When the rank range rod extends from the actual minimum to the actual maximum, it can be augmented by markings for the quartile ranks, including Q2 (median). This is shown for KeyRnks11 of the contingents in Fig. 7.12. Only the portions of the rods between Q1 and Q3 (the triangle pointers) were shown in Fig. 7.11. The diagram of Fig. 7.12 was generated by a special function facility named RankRods (Function 7.2). The RankRods function takes three inputs. The first input is an ordering vector like the OrderByQ1 vector used for Fig. 7.11. The second input is a data frame of the key ranks to be plotted. The third input is a vector that signals how each column of the data frame is to be handled in plotting, with each element signaling the respective column of the data frame. A zero, 0, indicates that the column is ignored in plotting. A −1 indicates that the column marks the lower ends of the ribs, and a 1 indicates that the column marks the upper ends of the ribs. A −2 indicates the column marker as an upward-pointing triangle, and a 2 indicates the column marker as a downward pointing triangle. A 3 indicates the column marker as a small circle.

After declaring KeyRnks11 to be a data frame, the instructions for generating Fig. 7.11 with this function are as follows:

```
@ Q1Q3rods <- c(0,-1,0,1,0)
@ OrderByQ1 <- rank(KeyRnks11[,2],ties.method="first")
@ RankRibs(OrderByQ1,KeyRnks11,Q1Q3rods)
@ identify(OrderByQ1,KeyRnks11[,2])
```

Function 7.2: RankRods Function for Plotting Augmented Rank Range Rods

```
RankRods <- function(Ordering,RpRnkFram,Ribbing)
{Ribs <- length(Ordering)
 # Ordering is an ordering vector for the ribs.
 # RpRnkFram is a data frame of representative ranks.
 # Ribbing controls rendering as follows—
 # 0 ignores a column
 # -1 is low end of rib and 1 is high end
 # -2 is upward triangle and 2 is downward triangle
 # 3 is a small circle
 RnkCols <- length(Ribbing)
 Riblo <- 1
 Ribhi <- RnkCols
 LoPnt <- 0
 HiPnt <- 0
 MidPnt <- 0
 for(I in 1:RnkCols)
  {if(Ribbing[I] == -1) Riblo <- I
   if(Ribbing[I] == 1) Ribhi <- I
   if(Ribbing[I] == -2) LoPnt <- I
   if(Ribbing[I] == 2) HiPnt <- I
   if(Ribbing[I] == 3) MidPnt <- I
  }
 MxRnk <- max(RpRnkFram[,Ribhi])
 plot(Ordering,RpRnkFram[,Riblo],ylim=c(0,MxRnk),ylab="Rank",pch=" ")
 for(I in 1:Ribs)
  {X <- c(Ordering[I],Ordering[I])
   Y <- c(RpRnkFram[I,Riblo],RpRnkFram[I,Ribhi])
   lines(X,Y)
  }
 if(HiPnt > 0)
  {for(I in 1:Ribs) points(Ordering[I],RpRnkFram[I,LoPnt],pch=2)
   for(I in 1:Ribs) points(Ordering[I],RpRnkFram[I,HiPnt],pch=6)
  }
 if(MidPnt > 0)
  for(I in 1:Ribs) points(Ordering[I],RpRnkFram[I,MidPnt])
}
```

Figure 7.12 was generated by the following set of **R** commands:

```
@ Ordering <- rank(KeyRnks11[,2],ties.method="first")
@ Rods <- c(-1,-2,3,2,1)
@ KeyRnks11 <- as.data.frame(KeyRnks11)
@ RankRods(Ordering,KeyRnks11,Rods)
@ identify(Ordering,KeyRnks11[,1])
```

Figure 7.12 shows that quartiles of representative ranks have substantial distinctiveness among the contingents, but minimum and maximum are relatively uninformative.

References

Brüggemann R, Patil GP (2010) Multicriteria prioritization and partial order in environmental sciences. Environ Ecol Stat 17(4):383–410

Brüggemann R, Welzl G, Voigt K (2003) Order theoretical tools for the evaluation of complex regional pollution patterns. J Chem Inf Comp Sci 43:1771–1779

Luther B, Brüggemann R, Pudenz S (2000) An approach to combine cluster analysis with order theoretical tools in problems of environmental pollution. Match 42:119–143

Mucha H (2002) Clustering techniques accompanied by matrix reordering techniques. In: Voigt K, Welzl G (eds) Order theoretical tools in environmental sciences – order theory (Hasse diagram technique) meets multivariate statistics. Shaker, Aachen, pp 129–140

Myers W, Patil GP (2010) Partial order and rank range runs for compositional complexes in landscape ecology and image analysis, with applications to restoration, remediation, and enhancement; Environmental and Ecological Statistics. In: 2010 JSM proceedings—statistics: a key to innovation in a data-centric world, Vancouver, BC, July 31–August 5, 2010. ISBN 978-0-9791747-9-7

Newlin J, Patil GP (2010) Application of partial order to bridge engineering, stream channel assessment, and infrastructure management. Environ Ecol Stat 17(4):437–454

Newlin J, Myers W, Patil GP, Joshi S (2010) Improving transparency of bridge condition for decision-making and analysis in bridge management. In: Frangopol D, Sause R, Kusko C (eds) Bridge maintenance, safety, management and life-cycle optimization. Taylor & Francis, London

Chapter 8
Case Comparisons and Precedence Pools

Having compared contingents on *constructed criteria* (centroids, representative ranks, and distance domains) to choose candidate contingents, our progressive prioritization process moves to comparison of cases within candidate contingents to choose candidate cases. Both comparison of contingents and comparison of cases within contingents can be seen as selective screening that eliminates cases from contention. This is followed by cross-contingent comparison of candidate cases that brings together the best cases of the better contingents. This combination of candidate cases that crosses contingents is then prioritized and particularized rather than reduced.

The quartiles of representative ranks (Figs. 7.3 and 7.4) have highlighted contingents 4, 5, and 7. Pairings of ORDITs from distance domains (Fig. 6.4) have highlighted contingents 7, 4, 6, and 10 if we include any contingent that received a 3 rating. Consolidation of PCO axis 1 across distance domains and consolidation of PCO axis 2 across distance domains (Fig. 7.6) have highlighted contingents 7, 4, 6, and 10. Integrating three views (Fig. 7.8) highlights contingents 7, 4, 6, and 10. Therefore, it seems practically prudent to conduct case comparisons for contingents 4, 5, 6, 7, and 10.

Conventional Criteria

Whereas constructed criteria were necessary for comparing contingents, case comparisons can be conducted on conventional criteria available as attributes (variates) from which contingents were configured by clustering. The product-order rating regime is completely comparative on a greater/lesser/same basis for each individual criterion. Therefore, comparisons conducted directly on the variate values as criteria yield the same result as comparisons of ranks—so ranking is optional.

W.L. Myers and G.P. Patil, *Multivariate Methods of Representing Relations in R for Prioritization Purposes*, Environmental and Ecological Statistics 6, DOI 10.1007/978-1-4614-3122-0_8, © Springer Science+Business Media, LLC 2012

However, ranks are preferred in subsequent steps, so the cases in each of these four contingents are isolated in terms of place-based ranks as follows:

```
@ Cntngn4 <- CasPlacRnk5[Klus11==4,]
@ Cntngn5 <- CasPlacRnk5[Klus11==5,]
@ Cntngn6 <- CasPlacRnk5[Klus11==6,]
@ Cntngn7 <- CasPlacRnk5[Klus11==7,]
@ Cntngn10 <- CasPlacRnk5[Klus11==10,]
@ length(Cntngn4[,1])
[1] 27
@ length(Cntngn5[,1])
[1] 33
@ length(Cntngn6[,1])
[1] 19
@ length(Cntngn7[,1])
[1] 17
@ length(Cntngn10[,1])
[1] 24
@ ID4 <- Cntngn4[,1]
@ ID5 <- Cntngn5[,1]
@ ID6 <- Cntngn6[,1]
@ ID7 <- Cntngn7[,1]
@ ID10 <- Cntngn10[,1]
```

The ProdOrdr function is then applied to each of these five contingents as follows:

```
@ ProdOrd4 <- ProdOrdr(ID4,Cntngn4[,-1],PlacBased)
@ ProdOrd5 <- ProdOrdr(ID5,Cntngn5[,-1],PlacBased)
@ ProdOrd6 <- ProdOrdr(ID6,Cntngn6[,-1],PlacBased)
@ ProdOrd7 <- ProdOrdr(ID7,Cntngn7[,-1],PlacBased)
@ ProdOrd10 <- ProdOrdr(ID10,Cntngn10[,-1],PlacBased)
```

A precedence plot for contingent 4 is shown in Fig. 8.1 with a companion progression plot in Fig. 8.2 according to the following sets of commands:

```
@ TrpzTrpl(ProdOrd4)
@ identify(ProdOrd4[,3],ProdOrd4[,2])

@ ORDITrank <- rank(ProdOrd4[,4])
@ ORDITstep <- rank(ProdOrd4[,4],ties.method="first")
@ plot(ORDITstep,ORDITrank)
@ identify(ORDITstep,ORDITrank)
```

The precedence plot is truncated on the right due to the maximum ascribed advantage being only a little over 30%. The limiting line is, thus, not shown in Fig. 8.1.

The identification numbers on the points are sequential line numbers in the data file. Therefore, they must be retrieved from the data file in order to determine the

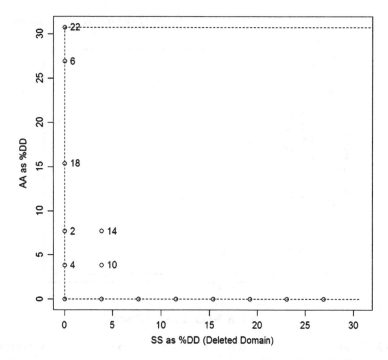

Fig. 8.1 Precedence plot of cases in contingent 4 based on ascribed advantage by product order for first five variates as indicators

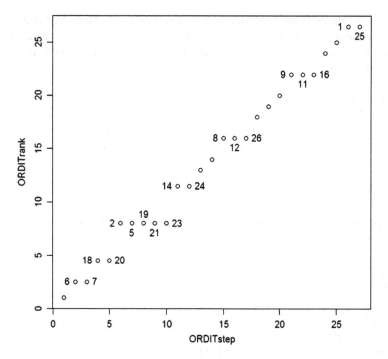

Fig. 8.2 Progression plot of cases in contingent 4 based on ascribed advantage by product order for first five variates as indicators

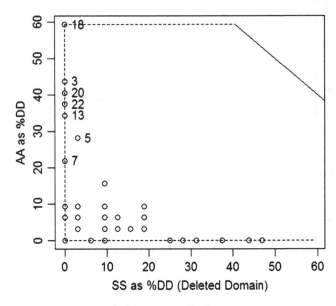

Fig. 8.3 Precedence plot of cases in contingent 5 based on ascribed advantage by product order for first five variates as indicators

hexagon ID numbers involved. The lines of hexagon data are retrieved in the order that they are listed for retrieval. Thus, hexagon 3268 occupies the 22nd line of the file for contingent 4. The numbers at the far left are line numbers in the parent CasPlacRnk5 file.

```
@ TopsOf4 <- c(22,6,7,18,20)
@ Cntngn4[TopsOf4,]
      HexID BirdSp MamlSp ElevSD PctFor Pct1FPch
120    3268  100.0   16.0   26.5      9      9.0
64     2647   36.0   63.0   12.0     26     26.5
65     2648   76.0    4.5   17.0     15     15.0
108    3141   89.5   34.5   55.5      2      2.0
110    3143   45.0   16.0   24.5     45     41.0
```

A precedence plot for contingent 5 is shown in Fig. 8.3 with its companion progression plot in Fig. 8.4.

```
@ TrpzTrpl(ProdOrd5)
@ identify(ProdOrd5[,3],ProdOrd5[,2])

@ ORDITrank <- rank(ProdOrd5[,4])
@ ORDITstep <- rank(ProdOrd5[,4],ties.method="first")
@ plot(ORDITstep,ORDITrank)
@ identify(ORDITstep,ORDITrank)
```

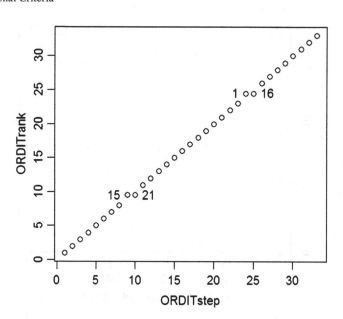

Fig. 8.4 Progression plot of cases in contingent 5 based on ascribed advantage by product order for first five variates as indicators

The progression plot shows no coincidence among the more conspicuous candidates in the precedence plot for contingent 5. This time, truncation leaves the upper part of the limiting line exposed.

Retrieval of the more conspicuous candidates proceeds as before.

```
@ TopsOf5 <- c(18,3,20,22,13,5,7)
@ Cntngn5[TopsOf5,]
     HexID BirdSp MamlSp ElevSD PctFor Pct1FPch
118  3266   18.0   16.0   92.0   24.5    24.0
19   2170   11.5   34.5  112.0   20.0    20.0
130  3393   18.0   63.0   90.0   18.0    18.0
142  3521   53.0   34.5  107.0    4.0     4.0
75   2769   76.0   34.5   86.0    9.0     9.0
30   2288   62.0   16.0   94.0   42.0    39.0
40   2405   76.0    8.5  100.5   21.5    21.5
```

A precedence plot for contingent 6 is shown in Fig. 8.5 with its companion progression plot in Fig. 8.6.

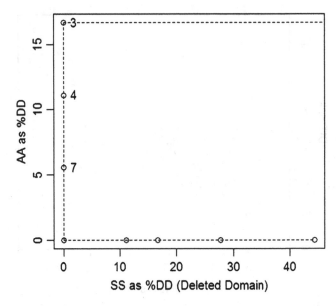

Fig. 8.5 Precedence plot of cases in contingent 6 based on ascribed advantage by product order for first five variates as indicators

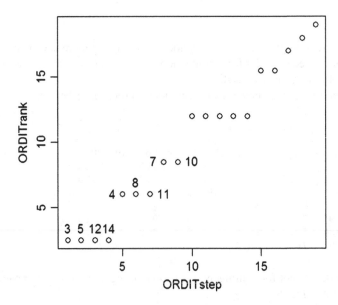

Fig. 8.6 Progression plot of cases in contingent 6 based on ascribed advantage by product order for first five variates as indicators

```
@ TrpzTrpl(ProdOrd6)
@ identify(ProdOrd6[,3],ProdOrd6[,2])

@ ORDITrank <- rank(ProdOrd6[,4])
@ ORDITstep <- rank(ProdOrd6[,4],ties.method="first")
@ plot(ORDITstep,ORDITrank)
@ identify(ORDITstep,ORDITrank)
```

As with contingent 4, the precedence plot for contingent 6 is truncated prior to the limiting line with maximum ascribed advantage being only a little more than 15%. There is strong coincidence in the precedence plot with four in the first position, three in the second position, and two in the third position.

The more conspicuous candidate cases for contingent 6 are retrieved as follows:

```
@ TopsOf6 <- c(3,5,12,14,4,8,11,7,10)
@ Cntngn6[TopsOf6,]
     HexID BirdSp MamlSp ElevSD PctFor Pct1FPch
34    2292    8.5  112.0   86.0  168.0    153.0
46    2411   45.0  138.5   78.5  157.5    146.0
93    2899  109.5  138.5   16.0  150.0    137.0
160   3657  109.5  127.5   28.0  142.0    140.0
42    2407   53.0   63.0   43.5  149.0    165.0
77    2771   25.0   91.0   78.5  170.5    150.5
82    2776   30.0  149.0   21.0  163.0    148.0
70    2653   45.0  149.0  123.0  140.0    158.0
81    2775   10.0  161.0   38.0  160.0    149.0
```

The precedence plot for contingent 7 appears in Fig. 8.7 with its companion progression plot in Fig. 8.8. There is extensive coincidence for this contingent, but it does not involve the only conspicuous candidate case.

```
@ TrpzTrpl(ProdOrd7)
@ identify(ProdOrd7[,3],ProdOrd7[,2])

@ ORDITrank <- rank(ProdOrd7[,4])
@ ORDITstep <- rank(ProdOrd7[,4],ties.method="first")
@ plot(ORDITstep,ORDITrank)
@ identify(ORDITstep,ORDITrank)

@ Cntngn7[15,]
     HexID BirdSp MamlSp ElevSD PctFor Pct1FPch
148   3527     30    4.5      9     68       66
```

Finally, the precedence plot for contingent 10 appears in Fig. 8.9 with its companion progression plot in Fig. 8.10.

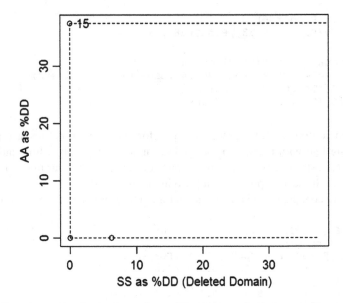

Fig. 8.7 Precedence plot of cases in contingent 7 based on ascribed advantage by product order for first five variates as indicators

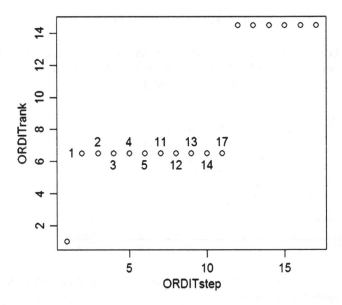

Fig. 8.8 Progression plot of cases in contingent 7 based on ascribed advantage by product order for first five variates as indicators

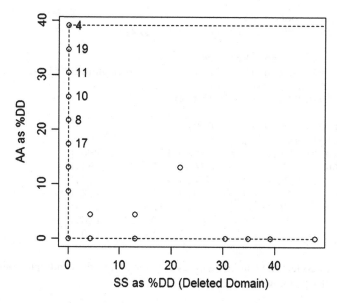

Fig. 8.9 Precedence plot of cases in contingent 10 based on ascribed advantage by product order for first five variates as indicators

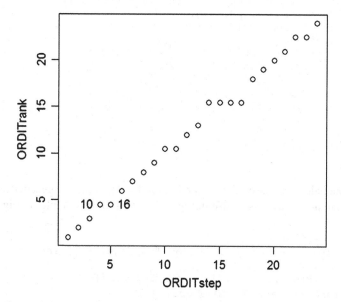

Fig. 8.10 Progression plot of cases in contingent 10 based on ascribed advantage by product order for first five variates as indicators

```
@ TrpzTrpl(ProdOrd10)
@ identify(ProdOrd10[,3],ProdOrd10[,2])

@ ORDITrank <- rank(ProdOrd10[,4])
@ ORDITstep <- rank(ProdOrd10[,4],ties.method="first")
@ plot(ORDITstep,ORDITrank)
@ identify(ORDITstep,ORDITrank)

@ TopsOf10 <- c(4,19,11,10,8,17)
@ Cntngn10[TopsOf10,]
     HexID BirdSp MamlSp ElevSD PctFor Pct1FPch
74    2768     62   63.0   74.5   96.0     94.5
147   3526     76   34.5   63.5  108.0    107.5
121   3269     45   34.5   90.0  109.0    122.0
114   3147     76   63.0   61.0  120.5    115.0
112   3145     53   16.0   61.0  130.5    126.0
144   3523     14   34.5  116.0  112.5    130.0
```

Next is to collect the candidate cases extracted from the candidate contingents, and then order them by HexID numbers.

```
@ Toppings <- rbind(Cntngn4[TopsOf4,],Cntngn5[TopsOf5,])
@ Toppings <- rbind(Toppings,Cntngn6[TopsOf6,])
@ Toppings <- rbind(Toppings,Cntngn7[15,])
@ Toppings <- rbind(Toppings,Cntngn10[TopsOf10,])
@ TopsOrdr <- order(Toppings[,1])
@ Toppings <- Toppings[TopsOrdr,]
@ head(Toppings)
    HexID BirdSp MamlSp ElevSD PctFor Pct1FPch
19   2170   11.5   34.5  112.0   20.0     20.0
30   2288   62.0   16.0   94.0   42.0     39.0
34   2292    8.5  112.0   86.0  168.0    153.0
40   2405   76.0    8.5  100.5   21.5     21.5
42   2407   53.0   63.0   43.5  149.0    165.0
46   2411   45.0  138.5   78.5  157.5    146.0
@ length(Toppings[,1])
[1] 28
```

We conclude this phase of the examination by determining precedence among these 28 candidate cases as shown in Fig. 8.11 with progression plot in Fig. 8.12.

```
@ IDtops <- Toppings[,1]
@ ProdOrdTops <- ProdOrdr(IDtops,Toppings[,-1],PlacBased)
@ TrpzTrpl(ProdOrdTops)
@ identify(ProdOrdTops[,3],ProdOrdTops[,2])
@ ORDITrank <- rank(ProdOrdTops[,4])
@ ORDITstep <- rank(ProdOrdTops[,4],ties.method="first")
@ plot(ORDITstep,ORDITrank)
@ identify(ORDITstep,ORDITrank)
```

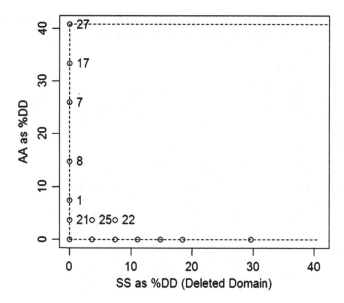

Fig. 8.11 Precedence plot for candidate cases

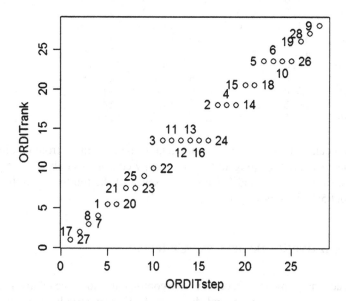

Fig. 8.12 Progression plot for candidate cases, labeled by sequence number

The progression plot of Fig. 8.12 is fully labeled by sequence number, and these are used to list the candidate cases in order of precedence.

```
@ TopsOrdr <- order(ProdOrdTops[,5])
@ Toppings[TopsOrdr,]
    HexID BirdSp MamlSp ElevSD PctFor Pct1FPch
148  3527   30.0    4.5    9.0   68.0     66.0
110  3143   45.0   16.0   24.5   45.0     41.0
64   2647   36.0   63.0   12.0   26.0     26.5
65   2648   76.0    4.5   17.0   15.0     15.0
19   2170   11.5   34.5  112.0   20.0     20.0
118  3266   18.0   16.0   92.0   24.5     24.0
120  3268  100.0   16.0   26.5    9.0      9.0
130  3393   18.0   63.0   90.0   18.0     18.0
144  3523   14.0   34.5  116.0  112.5    130.0
121  3269   45.0   34.5   90.0  109.0    122.0
34   2292    8.5  112.0   86.0  168.0    153.0
75   2769   76.0   34.5   86.0    9.0      9.0
77   2771   25.0   91.0   78.5  170.5    150.5
81   2775   10.0  161.0   38.0  160.0    149.0
108  3141   89.5   34.5   55.5    2.0      2.0
142  3521   53.0   34.5  107.0    4.0      4.0
30   2288   62.0   16.0   94.0   42.0     39.0
40   2405   76.0    8.5  100.5   21.5     21.5
82   2776   30.0  149.0   21.0  163.0    148.0
93   2899  109.5  138.5   16.0  150.0    137.0
112  3145   53.0   16.0   61.0  130.5    126.0
42   2407   53.0   63.0   43.5  149.0    165.0
46   2411   45.0  138.5   78.5  157.5    146.0
74   2768   62.0   63.0   74.5   96.0     94.5
147  3526   76.0   34.5   63.5  108.0    107.5
114  3147   76.0   63.0   61.0  120.5    115.0
160  3657  109.5  127.5   28.0  142.0    140.0
70   2653   45.0  149.0  123.0  140.0    158.0
```

The top candidate comes from contingent 7, the next three from contingent 4, and the next two from contingent 5. Contingent 7 contributes only the one premier candidate. Contingents 4 and 5 account for seven of the top ten, with the top ten being about 5% of the hexagons.

Representative Ranks as Case Criteria

Ascribed advantage by product order within contingent tends to be relatively limited, typically ranging between 15 and 40%. Product order strictly matches criteria between cases, and a small reversal of any criterion is sufficient to nullify advantage. Since the members of a contingent are chosen for similarity, small reversals of criteria are likely to occur. This is reflected in truncation of the limiting line and left-hand stacking as in Fig. 8.11 instead of diagonal decline as in Fig. 7.1. The strategy of using representative ranks can be applied at the case level by using specific order points from the rank distribution for each case. This relaxes the strict matching of criteria so that small reversals have less effect on the comparisons. Function 8.1 is a CasRnkos function that produces a data frame of five case rank order statistics comprising minimum (Min), first quartile (Q1), median (Q2), third quartile (Q3), and maximum (Max).

The CasRnkos function is applied to place-ranked data as follows:

```
@ CasRnkStat5 <- CasRnkos(CasPlacRnk5)
@ head(CasRnkStat5)
  CaseIDs RnkMin RnkQ1 RnkQ2 RnkQ3 RnkMax
1    1714    170 193.0 210.5 211.0  211.0
2    1827     67  69.0 190.5 205.0  210.0
3    1828    147 159.0 165.0 199.5  205.0
4    1829    187 202.0 202.5 208.0  210.5
5    1941      2   2.0 134.5 204.0  205.0
6    1942     92 106.5 148.0 179.0  187.0
```

Function 8.1: CasRnkos Function for Determining Rank Order Statistics of Cases

```
CasRnkos <- function (RankData)
# RankData is a data frame of place ranks with identifiers.
# Output is Min,Q1,Q2,Q3,Max by case.
{RnkCols <- length(RankData)
 Rnkcols <- RnkCols - 1
 Cases <- length(RankData[,1])
 RnkMin <- rep(0,Cases)
 RnkMax <- RnkMin
 RnkQ1 <- RnkMin
 RnkQ2 <- RnkMin
 RnkQ3 <- RnkMin
 for(I in 1:Cases)
  {CaseRnks <- rep(0,Rnkcols)
    for(J in 1:Rnkcols)
     {K <- J + 1
       CaseRnks[J] <- RankData[I,K]
     }
    RnkMin[I] <- min(CaseRnks)
    RnkMax[I] <- max(CaseRnks)
    RnkQ1[I] <- round(quantile(CaseRnks,probs=0.25),1)
    RnkQ2[I] <- round(median(CaseRnks),1)
    RnkQ3[I] <- round(quantile(CaseRnks,probs=0.75),1)
  }
 CaseIDs <- RankData[,1]
 CasRnkset <- cbind(CaseIDs,RnkMin,RnkQ1,RnkQ2,RnkQ3,RnkMax)
 CasRnkset <- as.data.frame(CasRnkset)
 CasRnkset
}
```

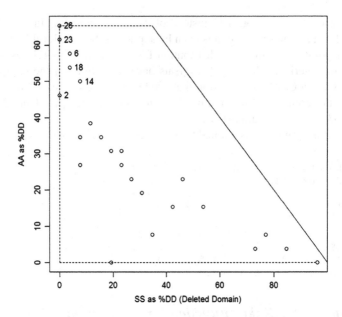

Fig. 8.13 Min–max (rank range) precedence plot for cases in contingent 4

The foregoing case screenings are next revisited using min–max and min–median–max as representative ranks. In so doing, precedence plots are done for min–max, whereas progression plots are replaced by plotting ranked ORDITs for min–median–max against ranked ORDITs for min–max. Preliminaries are as follows:

```
@ MnMx <- c(2,6)
@ MnMdMx <- c(2,4,6)
@ Cntngn4RR <- CasRnkStat5[Klus11==4,]
@ Cntngn5RR <- CasRnkStat5[Klus11==5,]
@ Cntngn6RR <- CasRnkStat5[Klus11==6,]
@ Cntngn7RR <- CasRnkStat5[Klus11==7,]
@ Cntngn10RR <- CasRnkStat5[Klus11==10,]
```

Operations for contingent 4 then proceed to obtain a min–max precedence plot shown in Fig. 8.13.

```
@ PrOr4MnMx <- ProdOrdr(ID4,Cntngn4RR[,MnMx],PlacBased)
@ PrOr4MnMdMx <- ProdOrdr(ID4,Cntngn4RR[,MnMdMx],PlacBased)
@ TrpzTrpl(PrOr4MnMx)
@ identify(PrOr4MnMx[,3],PrOr4MnMx[,2])
```

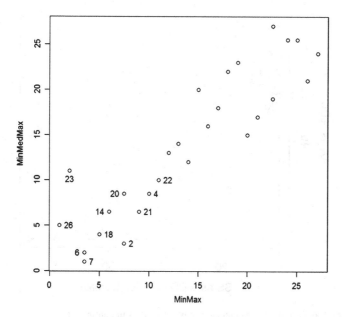

Fig. 8.14 Ranked ORDIT of min–median–max versus ranked ORDIT of min–max for contingent 4

The labeled cases in Fig. 8.13 are retrieved as follows:

```
@ TopRRof4 <- c(26,23,6,18,14,2)
@ Cntngn4RR[TopRRof4,]
    CaseIDs RnkMin RnkQ1 RnkQ2 RnkQ3 RnkMax
150    3529    1.5   45  48.0  55.5   76.0
126    3274   10.5   45  55.0  58.0   63.0
64     2647   12.0   26  26.5  36.0   63.0
108    3141    2.0    2  34.5  55.5   89.5
98     3017   13.0   43  51.0  53.0   63.0
20     2171   16.0   17  17.0  43.5   45.0
```

A cross-plot for min–median–max against min–max is then obtained and shown in Fig. 8.14.

```
@ plot(PrOr4MnMx[,5],PrOr4MnMdMx[,5],
@@ xlab="MinMax",ylab="MinMedMax")
@ identify(PrOr4MnMx[,5],PrOr4MnMdMx[,5])
```

Figure 8.14 shows that hexagon 2648 (7) is tied with hexagon 2647 (6) relative to min–max, and hexagon 3143 (20) is likewise tied with 2171 (2). The TopRRof4 is revised accordingly to reflect the ties. Figure 8.14 also shows that hexagon 3274 (23) has a median that is poorly placed relative to the ends of its range.

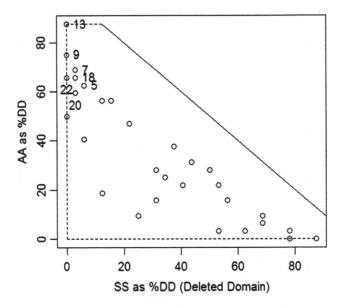

Fig. 8.15 Min–max (rank range) precedence plot for cases in contingent 5

```
@ Cntngn4RR[7,]
    CaseIDs RnkMin RnkQ1 RnkQ2 RnkQ3 RnkMax
65     2648    4.5    15    15    17    76
@ Cntngn4RR[20,]
     CaseIDs RnkMin RnkQ1 RnkQ2 RnkQ3 RnkMax
110    3143     16   24.5    41    45    45

@ TopRRof4 <- c(26,23,6,7,18,14,2,20)
```

Analysis for contingent 5 produces the precedence plot in Fig. 8.15.

```
@ PrOr5MnMx <- ProdOrdr(ID5,Cntngn5RR[,MnMx],PlacBased)
@ PrOr5MnMdMx <- ProdOrdr(ID5,Cntngn5RR[,MnMdMx],PlacBased)
@ TrpzTrpl(PrOr5MnMx)
@ identify(PrOr5MnMx[,3],PrOr5MnMx[,2])
```

A companion cross-plot for min–median–max against min–max is then obtained and shown in Fig. 8.16.

```
@ plot(PrOr5MnMx[,5],PrOr5MnMdMx[,5],
@@ xlab="MinMax",ylab="MinMedMax")
@ identify(PrOr5MnMx[,5],PrOr5MnMdMx[,5])
```

Figure 8.16 shows that item 21 is tied with item 20, and that hexagon 2526 (9) is anomalous with regard to inclusion of the median as a criterion.

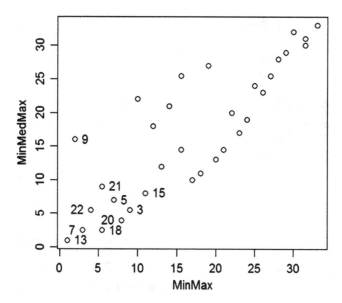

Fig. 8.16 Ranked ORDIT of min–median–max versus ranked ORDIT of min–max for contingent 5

```
@ Cntngn5RR[9,]
   CaseIDs RnkMin RnkQ1 RnkQ2 RnkQ3 RnkMax
53    2526    4.5  34.5    79    84    97
```

Hexagons highlighted from Figs. 8.15 and 8.16 are identified as follows:

```
@ TopRRof5 <- c(13,9,7,22,18,5,20,21)
@ Cntngn5RR[TopRRof5,]
    CaseIDs RnkMin RnkQ1 RnkQ2 RnkQ3 RnkMax
75     2769    9.0   9.0  34.5  76.0   86.0
53     2526    4.5  34.5  79.0  84.0   97.0
40     2405    8.5  21.5  21.5  76.0  100.5
142    3521    4.0   4.0  34.5  53.0  107.0
118    3266   16.0  18.0  24.0  24.5   92.0
30     2288   16.0  39.0  42.0  62.0   94.0
130    3393   18.0  18.0  18.0  63.0   90.0
141    3520   14.0  63.0  71.0  72.0   96.0
```

Hexagons 2170 (3) and 3015 (15) are also of interest in Fig. 8.16.

```
@ Cntngn5RR[c(3,15),]
   CaseIDs RnkMin RnkQ1 RnkQ2 RnkQ3 RnkMax
19    2170   11.5    20    20  34.5    112
96    3015   30.0    55    58  63.0     83
```

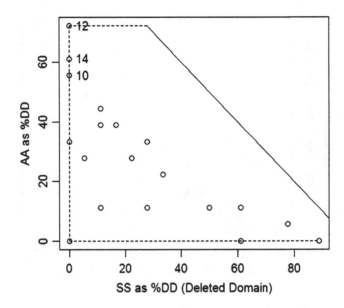

Fig. 8.17 Min–max (rank range) precedence plot for cases in contingent 6

Figure 8.17 shows the precedence plot for contingent 6 obtained as follows:

```
@ PrOr6MnMx <- ProdOrdr(ID6,Cntngn6RR[,MnMx],PlacBased)
@ PrOr6MnMdMx <- ProdOrdr(ID6,Cntngn6RR[,MnMdMx],PlacBased)
@ TrpzTrpl(PrOr6MnMx)
@ identify(PrOr6MnMx[,3],PrOr6MnMx[,2])
```

The companion cross-plot for min–median–max against min–max is shown in Fig. 8.18.

```
@ plot(PrOr6MnMx[,5],PrOr6MnMdMx[,5],
@@ xlab="MinMax",ylab="MinMedMax")
@ identify(PrOr6MnMx[,5],PrOr6MnMdMx[,5])
```

No concerns for ties arise from Fig. 8.18, but it does draw attention to two additional items. Including these two gives the following hexagons:

```
@ TopRRof6 <- c(12,14,10,5,7)
@ Cntngn6RR[TopRRof6,]
     CaseIDs RnkMin RnkQ1 RnkQ2 RnkQ3 RnkMax
93      2899     16 109.5 137.0 138.5  150.0
160     3657     28 109.5 127.5 140.0  142.0
81      2775     10  38.0 149.0 160.0  161.0
46      2411     45  78.5 138.5 146.0  157.5
70      2653     45 123.0 140.0 149.0  158.0
```

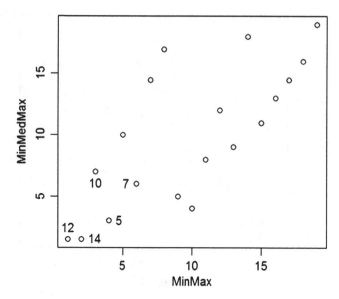

Fig. 8.18 Ranked ORDIT of min–median–max versus ranked ORDIT of min–max for contingent 6

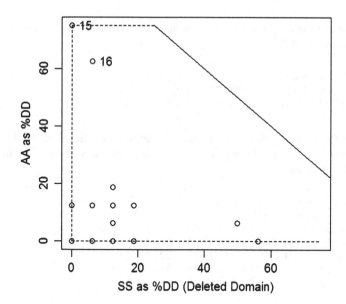

Fig. 8.19 Min–max (rank range) precedence plot for cases in contingent 7

The scenario for contingent 7 gives the precedence plot in Fig. 8.19.

```
@ PrOr7MnMx <- ProdOrdr(ID7,Cntngn7RR[,MnMx],PlacBased)
@ PrOr7MnMdMx <- ProdOrdr(ID7,Cntngn7RR[,MnMdMx],PlacBased)
@ TrpzTrpl(PrOr7MnMx)
@ identify(PrOr7MnMx[,3],PrOr7MnMx[,2])
```

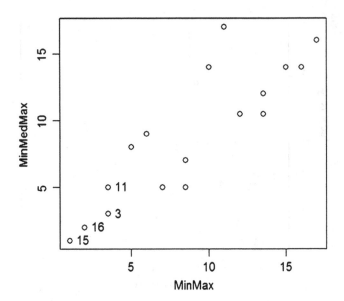

Fig. 8.20   Ranked ORDIT of min–median–max versus ranked ORDIT of min–max for contingent 7

The companion cross-plot of min–median–max against min–max for contingent 7 is shown in Fig. 8.20.

```
@ plot(PrOr7MnMx[,5],PrOr7MnMdMx[,5],
@@ xlab="MinMax",ylab="MinMedMax")
@ identify(PrOr7MnMx[,5],PrOr7MnMdMx[,5])
```

Although the items identified in Fig. 8.19 do not have ties, Fig. 8.20 indicates that the tied items 3 and 11 might also be of interest. Accordingly, the items are identified as follows:

```
@ TopRRof7 <- c(15,16,3,11)
@ Cntngn7RR[TopRRof7,]
     CaseIDs RnkMin RnkQ1 RnkQ2 RnkQ3 RnkMax
148     3527    4.5   9.0  30.0  66.0   68.0
149     3528    4.5  32.0  36.0 102.0  104.5
43      2408   15.0  16.0  21.5  91.0  112.0
123     3271    8.0  34.5  76.0 112.5  117.5
```

Exploration of contingents at the case level concludes with contingent 10, for which the precedence plot appears in Fig. 8.21.

```
@ PrOr10MnMx <- ProdOrdr(ID10,Cntngn10RR[,MnMx],PlacBased)
@ PrOr10MnMdMx <- ProdOrdr(ID10,Cntngn10RR[,MnMdMx],PlacBased)
@ TrpzTrpl(PrOr10MnMx)
@ identify(PrOr10MnMx[,3],PrOr10MnMx[,2])
```

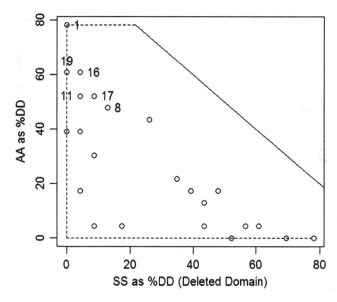

Fig. 8.21 Min–max (rank range) precedence plot for cases in contingent 10

The companion cross-plot of min–median–max against min–max for contingent 10 appears in Fig. 8.22 showing that item 17 is not as well situated when the median is also considered.

```
@ plot(PrOr10MnMx[,5],PrOr10MnMdMx[,5],
@@ xlab="MinMax",ylab="MinMedMax")
@ identify(PrOr10MnMx[,5],PrOr10MnMdMx[,5])
```

The labeled cases for contingent 10 are identified as follows:

```
@ TopRRof10 <- c(1,19,16,11,8,17)
@ Cntngn10RR[TopRRof10,]
```

	CaseIDs	RnkMin	RnkQ1	RnkQ2	RnkQ3	RnkMax
33	2291	1.5	74.5	99.0	106.5	127.5
147	3526	34.5	63.5	76.0	107.5	108.0
138	3401	4.5	25.0	77.0	120.0	128.5
121	3269	34.5	45.0	90.0	109.0	122.0
112	3145	16.0	53.0	61.0	126.0	130.5
144	3523	14.0	34.5	112.5	116.0	130.0

Finally, we pool the items of interest from the respective contingents and prepare a pooled precedence plot which appears in Fig. 8.23. Although we ordered the pool for conventional criteria by hexagon number, it is not really necessary to do so.

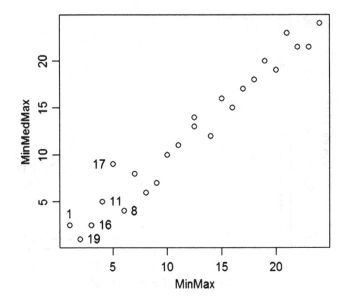

Fig. 8.22 Ranked ORDIT of min–median–max versus ranked ORDIT of min–max for contingent 10

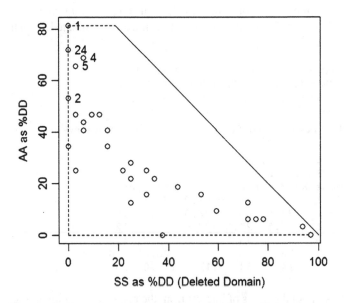

Fig. 8.23 Min–max (rank range) precedence plot for pooled items of interest

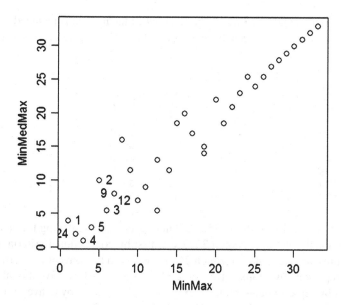

Fig. 8.24 Ranked ORDIT of min–median–max versus ranked ORDIT of min–max for contingent pooled items of interest

```
@ TopRR <- rbind(Cntngn4RR[TopRRof4,],Cntngn5RR[TopRRof5,])
@ TopRR <- rbind(TopRR,Cntngn5RR[c(3,15),])
@ TopRR <- rbind(TopRR,Cntngn6RR[TopRRof6,])
@ TopRR <- rbind(TopRR,Cntngn7RR[TopRRof7,])
@ TopRR <- rbind(TopRR,Cntngn10RR[TopRRof10,])
@ length(TopRR[,1])
[1] 33
@ IDTopRR <- TopRR[,1]

@ PrOrTopRRMnMx <- ProdOrdr(IDTopRR,TopRR[,MnMx],PlacBased)
@ PrOrTopRRMnMdMx <- ProdOrdr(IDTopRR,TopRR[,MnMdMx],PlacBased)
@ TrpzTrpl(PrOrTopRRMnMx)
@ identify(PrOrTopRRMnMx[,3],PrOrTopRRMnMx[,2])
```

The companion cross-plot of min–median–max against min–max for pooled items of interest appears in Fig. 8.24.

```
@ plot(PrOrTopRRMnMx[,5],PrOrTopRRMnMdMx[,5],
@@ xlab="MinMax",ylab="MinMedMax")
@ identify(PrOrTopRRMnMx[,5],PrOrTopRRMnMdMx[,5])
```

The top four candidate cases are the same when the median is included, but some shifts show in the next four. Selective retrieval of these candidate cases is as follows:

```
@ Top8byRR <- c(1,24,4,5,3,9,2,12)
@ TopRR[Top8byRR,]
    CaseIDs RnkMin RnkQ1 RnkQ2 RnkQ3 RnkMax
150    3529    1.5     45  48.0  55.5   76.0
148    3527    4.5      9  30.0  66.0   68.0
65     2648    4.5     15  15.0  17.0   76.0
108    3141    2.0      2  34.5  55.5   89.5
64     2647   12.0     26  26.5  36.0   63.0
75     2769    9.0      9  34.5  76.0   86.0
126    3274   10.5     45  55.0  58.0   63.0
142    3521    4.0      4  34.5  53.0  107.0
```

It is noteworthy that hexagon 3529 did not appear after screening for precedence by conventional criteria. Hexagon 3527 was first by conventional criteria and second by representative ranks. Hexagon 2648 was fourth by conventional criteria and third by representative ranks. Hexagon 3141 was 15th by conventional criteria and fourth by representative ranks. Hexagon 2647 was third by conventional criteria and fifth by representative ranks. Hexagon 2769 was 12th by conventional criteria and sixth by representative ranks. Hexagon 3274 did not appear after screening for precedence by conventional criteria. Hexagon 3521 was 12th by conventional criteria and eighth by representative ranks.

There is, thus, considerable consensus with regard to precedence for hexagons 3527, 2648, and 2647. Hexagons 2647 and 2648 are adjoining in the northeast corner of the state, whereas hexagon 3527 is located in the southwest corner of the state. Hexagon 2769 is adjacent to 2647 and 2648. Only one hexagon separates 3527 from 3529 and 3274.

Partial Precedence Pools

After having formed a pool of items of interest (candidate cases) drawn from different contingents, it may be appropriate to have a preliminary partitioning of the pool into partial precedence pools (Myers and Patil 2008). This would generally not be as advisable for earlier stages of screening due to computational considerations since it is not a local modeling approach that can avoid cumbersome combinatorial computation at the outset (Jones et al. 2009).

Partial precedence pools are based on ideas of domination and subordination according to product-order protocols, but focus on aggregate relations among subsets rather than precedence in pairs. Ascribed advantage and subordinate status by product-order relations provide the point of departure. One instance dominates another if it has ascribed advantage by the product-order protocols introduced earlier. Reciprocally, an instance is subordinate to another if the other has ascribed advantage by the product-order protocol, that is, the sense in which one instance dominates another if it is at least as good on all indicators and better on at least one indicator with an instance being subordinate to another if it is dominated by that other instance. We proceed to use these ideas for progressively partitioning a pool of instances into subsets (partial precedence pools) that have a sense of aggregate ordering (sequenced sets) with regard to dominance and subordination. The partition is done in two modes, and then the intersections of the two sets of subsets are considered with regard to joint ordering.

We first do progressive partitioning into what we call subordination steps and abbreviate as *SubSteps*, whereby each successive step has a stronger sense of being subordinate. This progressive process proceeds through a series of levels of elimination. It begins with all of the instances in a single pool, and segregates all of the instances that are not dominated by any other instances. The nondominated instances are placed in a partial pool that is numbered zero (0) since there is no (zero) domination of these instances. The pool of remaining instances has a least some domination by (some of) those in the initial partial pool. The process then repeats in progressive (recursive) fashion by isolating those in the (remaining) pool that are not dominated by any others in the (remaining) pool. This second partial pool is assigned level one (1) since its members are subject to one level of domination (by those in the zero-level partial pool). This recursion continues until the (residual) pool has no members that are dominated by any others in the (residual) pool. That final (residual) pool receives the highest level number since its degree of being dominated has persisted through the most stages of elimination. In precedence plots, SubStep level number is used as the SS axis replacing subordinate status based on percentage frequency in the deleted domain of other instances. It should also be noted that one extremely good indicator is sufficient to place an instance in the zero-level partial pool since it precludes domination of that instance even if other indicators are inferior. Thus, the zero-level partial pool may contain many mixed messages along with those that are more uniformly favorable.

A complementary process of progressive partial pools reflects capacity to dominate other instances rather than focusing on not being dominated. Dominating is done by way of superiority with no assistance from mixed messages. This process of determining dominance as aggregate advantage (Agrg8Adv) begins by segregating all of the instances in the general pool that do not dominate anything else. These are assigned to level zero (0) since they have no dominating capacity. The instances which dominate something else in the pool remain in the pool for further consideration in the next round of recursion. After segregating all of the level zero instances as a zero-numbered partial pool, the process repeats by finding those among the remainder that do not dominate anything in the current pool and assigning them to level one (1) since they have aggregate advantage only at the initial level. The process continues recursively through additional levels of partial pooling until a residual pool is reached that contains no domination. The final residual pool receives the highest level number since its members have retained dominating capability up to this ultimate level. The numbering is, thus, according to differences in "depth of dominating". This level number is used in precedence plots as the AA axis replacing ascribed advantage based on percentage frequency of advantage in the deleted domain of competing cases.

Partitioning into SS subordination steps is accomplished by Function 8.2 named SubSteps. It takes three inputs, with the first being a data frame of indicators. The second is a vector of status numbers for the instances. A nonnegative status number indicates that the analysis is conducted one level at a time, with all of the nonnegative status numbers being processed in previous passes and current level number to begin with the available nonnegative number. This provision is made because computations are computationally cumbersome and become time consuming for large numbers of instances. If all negative numbers are −1, then the process will transpire to completion in the current run. If all negative status numbers are −2 or less, then only one level of elimination will take place in the current pass. The third input indicates whether (1) or not (0) the indicators are of a place-based nature.

Function 8.2: SubSteps Function for Determining Partial Pools of SS Levels

```
SubSteps <- function(Ratings,Status,Placing)
{LastLvl <- max(Status)
 if(LastLvl < 0) LastLvl <- -1
 MinStatus <- min(Status)
 Ncol <- length(Ratings)
 Ncase <- length(Ratings[,1])
 Undone <- 0
 for(I in 1:Ncase) if(Status[I] < 0) Undone <- Undone + 1
 Levl <- LastLvl
 Asignd <- 0
 while(Asignd < Undone)
  {for(I in 1:Ncase)
    {if(Status[I]<0)
      {Undom <- 1
        for(J in 1:Ncase)
         {if(Status[J]<0 | Status[J]>Levl)
            {MatchA <- 0; MatchB <- 0
             VecA <- Ratings[I,] - Ratings[J,]
             if(Placing>0) VecA <- Ratings[J,] - Ratings[I,]
             if(max(VecA) > 0) MatchA <- 1
             if(min(VecA) < 0) MatchB <- 1
             if(MatchA==0 & MatchB==1) Undom <- 0
            }
         }
        if(Undom==1)
         {Status[I] <- (Levl+1)
          Asignd <- (Asignd+1)
         }
      }
    }
   Levl <- (Levl+1)
   if(MinStatus < -1) Asignd <- Undone
  }
 Status
}
```

Partitioning into AA levels of aggregate advantage is accomplished by the Agrg8Adv Function 8.3, for which inputs are the same as for the SubSteps Function 8.2.

Function 8.3: Agrg8Adv Function for Determining Partial Pools of AA Levels

```
Agrg8Adv <- function(Ratings,Status,Placing)
{LastLvl <- max(Status)
 if(LastLvl < 0) LastLvl <- -1
 MinStatus <- min(Status)
 Ncol <- length(Ratings)
 Ncase <- length(Ratings[,1])
 Undone <- 0
 for(I in 1:Ncase) if(Status[I] < 0) Undone <- Undone + 1
 Levl <- LastLvl
 Asignd <- 0
 while(Asignd < Undone)
  {for(I in 1:Ncase)
    {if(Status[I] < 0)
      {Nosub <- 1
        for(J in 1:Ncase)
         {if(Status[J]<0 | Status[J]>Levl)
            {MatchA <- 0; MatchB <- 0
             VecA <- Ratings[I,] - Ratings[J,]
             if(Placing>0) VecA <- Ratings[J,] - Ratings[I,]
             if(max(VecA) > 0) MatchA <- 1
             if(min(VecA) < 0) MatchB <- 1
             if(MatchA==1 & MatchB==0) Nosub <- 0
            }
         }
        if(Nosub==1)
         {Status[I] <- (Levl+1)
          Asignd <- (Asignd+1)
         }
      }
    }
   Levl <- (Levl+1)
   if(MinStatus < -1) Asignd <- Undone
  }
 Status
}
```

For the Toppings pool based on conventional criteria with precedence plot in Fig. 8.9 and incidence plot in Fig. 8.10, SS levels are obtained as follows:

```
@ ToppingSS <- rep(-1,28)
@ ToppingSS <- SubSteps(Toppings[,-1],ToppingSS,PlacBased)
@ max(ToppingSS)
[1] 2
```

Thus, the cases in the Toppings pool have segregated into three SS levels inclusive of the zero level. AA levels are obtained in like manner.

```
@ ToppingAA <- rep(-1,28)
@ ToppingAA <- Agrg8Adv(Toppings[,-1],ToppingAA,PlacBased)
@ max(ToppingAA)
[1] 2
```

Having determined the SS and AA levels, the PrtlPool Function 8.4 is used to compute ORDITs. In this mode, the ranked ORDITs are called "placements."

```
@ ToppingOrd <- PrtlPool(Toppings[,1],ToppingAA,ToppingSS)
@ head(ToppingOrd)
  CaseIDs AA SS ORDIT Placment
1    2170  2  0   0.0      2.0
2    2288  0  1   2.5     22.0
3    2292  0  0   2.0     13.5
4    2405  0  1   2.5     22.0
5    2407  0  1   2.5     22.0
```

Function 8.4: PrtlPool Function for Determining ORDITs of Partial Pools

```
PrtlPool <- function(CaseIDs,AA,SS)
{Cases <- length(CaseIDs)
 MaxAA <- max(AA)
 MaxSS <- max(SS)
# CCC is condition complement component as MaxAA - AA
# BBB is bipartite basal bar component as a decimal fraction
 CCC <- rep(0,Cases)
 BBB <- CCC
 ORDIT <- CCC
 for(I in 1:Cases)
  {CCC[I] <- MaxAA - AA[I]
   if(AA[I] < MaxAA) BBB[I] <- SS[I]/MaxSS
   if(BBB[I] > 0.999) BBB[I] <- 0.999
   BBB[I] <- round(BBB[I],digits=3)
   ORDIT[I] <- CCC[I]+BBB[I]
  }
 Placment <- rank(ORDIT)
 Placement <- cbind(CaseIDs,AA,SS,ORDIT,Placment)
 Placement <- as.data.frame(Placement)
 Placement
}
```

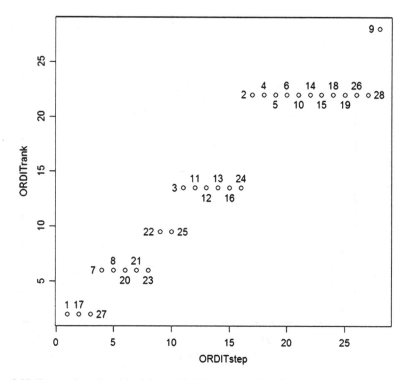

Fig. 8.25 Progression plot of partial pools for Toppings pool based on conventional criteria

A progression plot can then be obtained as follows and shown in Fig. 8.25:

```
@ ORDITrank <- rank(ToppingOrd[,4])
@ ORDITstep <- rank(ToppingOrd[,4],ties.method="first")
@ plot(ORDITstep,ORDITrank)
@ identify(ORDITstep,ORDITrank)
```

The progression plot in Fig. 8.25 shows six partial pools. The hexagons in the first (best) partial pool are retrieved as follows:

```
@ Toppings[c(1,17,27),]
19    2170    11.5    34.5    112.0    20    20
110   3143    45.0    16.0     24.5    45    41
148   3527    30.0     4.5      9.0    68    66
```

The hexagons in the second best partial pool are obtained likewise.

```
@ Toppings[c(7,8,20,21,23),]
     HexID  BirdSp  MamlSp  ElevSD  PctFor  Pct1FPch
64    2647      36    63.0    12.0    26.0      26.5
65    2648      76     4.5    17.0    15.0      15.0
118   3266      18    16.0    92.0    24.5      24.0
120   3268     100    16.0    26.5     9.0       9.0
130   3393      18    63.0    90.0    18.0      18.0
```

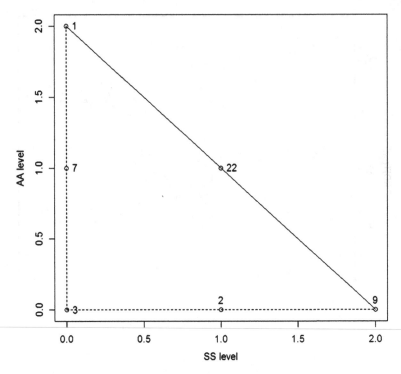

Fig. 8.26 Precedence plot for partial pools by conventional criteria. Each point label identifies a representative member of the partial pool as shown in the progression plot of Fig. 8.25

The PoolPlot Function 8.5 generates a precedence plot for partial pools. This is applied as follows and shown in Fig. 8.26:

```
@ PoolPlot(ToppingOrd)
@ identify(ToppingOrd[,3],ToppingOrd[,2])
```

Each point label in the precedence plot identifies a representative member of the partial pool as shown in the incidence plot of Fig. 8.25. For example, the third partial pool on the center of the diagonal limiting line is as follows:

```
@ Toppings[c(22,25),]
    HexID BirdSp MamlSp ElevSD PctFor Pct1FPch
121  3269     45   34.5     90  109.0      122
144  3523     14   34.5    116  112.5      130
```

The partial pool with the most conflicts in the criteria is situated at the lower-left corner of the precedence plot.

```
@ Toppings[c(3,11,12,13,16,24),]
    HexID BirdSp MamlSp ElevSD PctFor Pct1FPch
34   2292    8.5  112.0   86.0  168.0   153.0
75   2769   76.0   34.5   86.0    9.0     9.0
77   2771   25.0   91.0   78.5  170.5   150.5
81   2775   10.0  161.0   38.0  160.0   149.0
108  3141   89.5   34.5   55.5    2.0     2.0
142  3521   53.0   34.5  107.0    4.0     4.0
```

Function 8.5: PoolPlot Facility for Generating Precedence Plots for Partial Pools

```
PoolPlot <- function(Placement)
# Input is data frame of partial pool placements.
{Cases <- length(Placement[,1])
 Ymax <- max(Placement[,2])
 Ymin <- min(Placement[,2])
 Xmax <- max(Placement[,3])
 Xmin <- min(Placement[,3])
 Xright <- Ymax
 if(Xmax > Ymax) Xright <- Xmax
 plot(Placement[,3],Placement[,2],ylab="AA level",
  xlab="SS level",xlim=c(0,Xright))
 YY <- c(Ymax,Ymin)
 XX <- c(Xmin,Ymax)
 lines(XX,YY,lty=1)
 XX <- c(Xmin,Xmin)
 YY <- c(Ymin,Ymax)
 lines(XX,YY,lty=2)
 XX <- c(Xmin,Ymax)
 if(Xmax > Ymax) XX <- c(Xmin,Xmax)
 YY <- c(Ymin,Ymin)
 lines(XX,YY,lty=2)
 XX <- c(Xmin,Ymin)
 YY <- c(Ymax,Ymax)
 lines(XX,YY,lty=2)
}
```

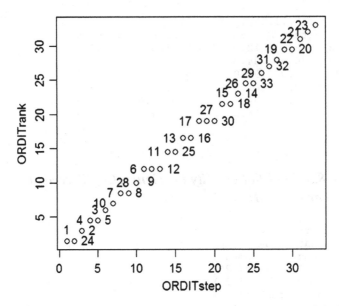

Fig. 8.27 Progression plot of partial pools for TopRR pool based on rank range (Min–Max)

Pursuing partial pools in terms of representative ranks concludes this chapter on case comparatives. The pool from representative ranks is in TopRR. For rank range (MnMx), this is accomplished as follows:

```
@ TopRRSS <- rep(-1,33)
@ TopRRSS <- SubSteps(TopRR[,MnMx],TopRRSS,PlacBased)
@ max(TopRRSS)
[1] 9
@ TopRRAA <- rep(-1,33)
@ TopRRAA <- Agrg8Adv(TopRR[,MnMx],TopRRAA,PlacBased)
@ max(TopRRAA)
[1] 9
@ TopRRord <- PrtlPool(TopRR[,1],TopRRAA,TopRRSS)
```

A progression plot is generated as follows and appears in Fig. 8.27:

```
@ ORDITrank <- rank(TopRRord[,4])
@ ORDITstep <- rank(TopRRord[,4],ties.method="first")
@ plot(ORDITstep,ORDITrank)
@ identify(ORDITstep,ORDITrank)
```

It is seen from Fig. 8.27 that the partial pools are numerous and small, containing only one, two, or three cases. Cases in the first seven pools are as follows:

```
@ TopRR[c(1,24),]
    CaseIDs RnkMin RnkQ1 RnkQ2 RnkQ3 RnkMax
150    3529    1.5    45    48  55.5     76
148    3527    4.5     9    30  66.0     68

@ TopRR[2,]
    CaseIDs RnkMin RnkQ1 RnkQ2 RnkQ3 RnkMax
126    3274   10.5    45    55    58     63

@ TopRR[c(4,5),]
    CaseIDs RnkMin RnkQ1 RnkQ2 RnkQ3 RnkMax
65     2648    4.5    15  15.0  17.0   76.0
108    3141    2.0     2  34.5  55.5   89.5

@ TopRR[3,]
   CaseIDs RnkMin RnkQ1 RnkQ2 RnkQ3 RnkMax
64    2647     12    26  26.5    36     63

@ TopRR[10,]
   CaseIDs RnkMin RnkQ1 RnkQ2 RnkQ3 RnkMax
53    2526    4.5  34.5    79    84     97

@ TopRR[c(7,8),]
    CaseIDs RnkMin RnkQ1 RnkQ2 RnkQ3 RnkMax
```

A partial pool precedence plot for rank range is obtained as follows and shown in Fig. 8.28, with the labeling numbers again being a representative of the partial pool:

```
@ PoolPlot(TopRRord)
@ identify(TopRRord[,3],TopRRord[,2])
```

The corresponding pooled precedence perspective for Min–Median–Max is obtained as follows, with progression plot in Fig. 8.29:

```
@ TopRRSSmmm <- rep(-1,33)
@ TopRRSSmmm <- SubSteps(TopRR[,MnMdMx],TopRRSSmmm,PlacBased)
@ max(TopRRSSmmm)
[1] 6
@ TopRRAAmmm <- rep(-1,33)
@ TopRRAAmmm <- Agrg8Adv(TopRR[,MnMdMx],TopRRAAmmm,PlacBased)
@ max(TopRRAAmmm)
[1] 6
@ TopRRordmmm <- PrtlPool(TopRR[,1],TopRRAAmmm,TopRRSSmmm)
@ ORDITrank <- rank(TopRRordmmm[,4])
@ ORDITstep <- rank(TopRRordmmm[,4],ties.method="first")
@ plot(ORDITstep,ORDITrank)
@ identify(ORDITstep,ORDITrank)
```

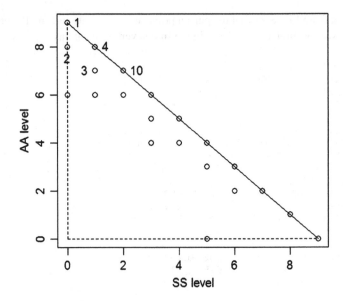

Fig. 8.28 Precedence plot for partial pools by rank range

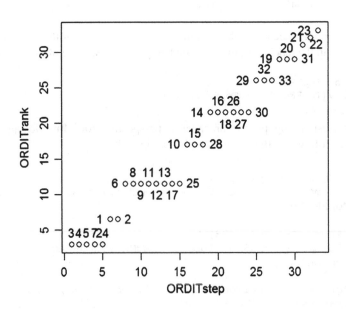

Fig. 8.29 Progression plot of partial pools for TopRR pool based on (Min–Median–Max)

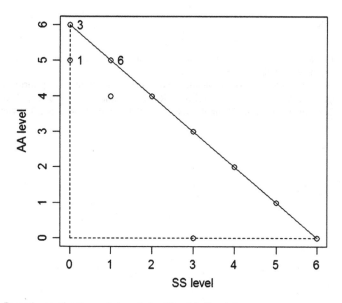

Fig. 8.30 Precedence plot for partial pools by Min–Median–Max

```
@ TopRR[c(3,4,5,7,24),]
     CaseIDs RnkMin RnkQ1 RnkQ2 RnkQ3 RnkMax
64      2647   12.0    26  26.5  36.0   63.0
65      2648    4.5    15  15.0  17.0   76.0
108     3141    2.0     2  34.5  55.5   89.5
20      2171   16.0    17  17.0  43.5   45.0
148     3527    4.5     9  30.0  66.0   68.0

@ TopRR[c(1,2),]
     CaseIDs RnkMin RnkQ1 RnkQ2 RnkQ3 RnkMax
150     3529    1.5    45    48  55.5     76
126     3274   10.5    45    55  58.0     63
```

It can be seen that the additional criterion has resulted in fewer (and therefore
larger) pools, which is typical. The partial pool precedence plot for Min–Median–
Max is given in Fig. 8.30.

```
@ PoolPlot(TopRRordmmm)
@ identify(TopRRordmmm[,3],TopRRordmmm[,2])
```

Hexagons 3527, 2647, and 2648 are again prominent across the pooled
comparisons.

References

Jones O, Maillardet R, Robinson A (2009) Introduction to scientific programming and simulation with R. Chapman & Hall/CRC, Boca Raton, FL

Myers W, Patil GP (2008) Semi-subordination sequences in multi-measure prioritization problems, chap. 7. In: Pavan M, Todeschini R (eds) Ranking methods: theory and applications, vol. 27, data handling in science and technology. Elsevier Publishing, Amsterdam, The Netherlands, pp 159–168

Chapter 9
Distal Data and Indicator Interactions

Although representative ranks are indirect indicators with intrinsic indefiniteness, they are particularly advantageous for determining whether there are cases having pronounced sensitivity to a change in one indicator. It may be that one indicator has especially good status, whereby deterioration in the indicator would degrade the overall status of the case substantially. Conversely, it may be that an indicator has especially poor status, whereby improvement in the indicator would upgrade the overall status of the case substantially. In the latter situation, some remediation effort focused on the weak indicator could pay large dividends (Newlin and Bhat 2007). Statistically, a sensitive situation involves a rank outlier producing an extended tail on the distribution of ranks for the case, which can occur on one or both ends.

Even though indicators appear to be substantially correlated in an overall sense, the presence of additional indicators may reveal atypical cases that are expressed in what may be considered "indicator interaction." Whereas two indicators may typically track each other closely, they may depart noticeably from that pattern for particular cases. This interplay of indicators is signaling that the cases cannot all be covered with a broad brush. Those cases that show as anomalies in the joint pattern must be examined individually to find the features that are inducing the interplay. This chapter is concerned with irregularities in ranks that reveal the need for extended explorations of etiology.

Distal Data and End Extensions

Consider the row of (place based) ranks for a case being sorted in ascending order. Let the (numerically) largest rank be the *major maximum* and the second largest be the *minor maximum*, these being the *upper extremities*. If there are ties for major, the major and minor are same. Let the least rank be the *major minimum* and the

Fig. 9.1 Diagrammatic
representation of extremity
extents

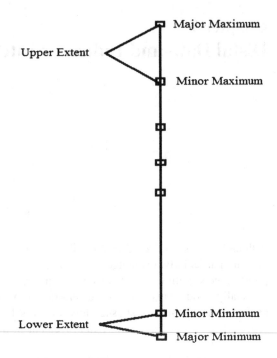

second least be the *minor minimum*, these being the *lower extremities*. Let the
upper extent ($\dot{m}$) be defined as the difference between the major maximum and
the minor maximum:

$$\text{upper extent } (\dot{m}) = \text{major maximum} - \text{minor maximum}$$

Also let the lower extent (m) be defined as the difference between the major minimum and the minor minimum:

$$\text{lower extent } (\underset{\cdot}{m}) = \text{major minimum} - \text{minor minimum}$$

For major ties, the respective extent is taken to be 0. Note that upper extent has
a positive sense and lower extent has a negative sense. Figure 9.1 is a diagrammatic
representation of the extremity extents.

A large value of $\dot{m}$ indicates that a particular criterion is substantially degrading
status for the case, making it a candidate for single-criterion remediation. A numerically large value of m indicates that a particular criterion is substantially elevating
status for the case, making it a candidate for a retention regime. Small or moderate
extremity extents indicate that no single criterion is critical for the case.

Based on extremity extents, we proceed to create a distal (farthest from the middle) dataset. For each case, determine $\dot{m}$ and m and identify the criteria in the major
positions. Assign a value of 0 for all criteria (indicators) not in a major position.

Assign m to the criterion in major minimum position. Assign $\dot{m}$ to the criterion in major maximum position. Function 9.1 called Xtremity serves to determine a distal dataset from a data frame of place ranks having Case ID number in the first column.

Function 9.1: Xtremity Function Facility for Determining Distal Data from Ranks

```
Xtremity <- function(RankData)
# RankData is a data frame of place ranks with CaseID in first column.
{RnkCols <- length(RankData)
 Rnkcols <- RnkCols -1
 Cases <- length(RankData[,1])
 XtrmXtnt <- RankData
 for(I in 1:Cases)
  {CaseRnks <- rep(0,Rnkcols)
    for(J in 1:Rnkcols)
     {K <- J + 1
      CaseRnks[J] <- RankData[I,K]
     }
   MinRnk <- min(CaseRnks)
   MaxRnk <- max(CaseRnks)
   Maxx <- 0
   Minn <- 0
   for(J in 1:Rnkcols)
    {if(CaseRnks[J]>=MaxRnk) Maxx <- J
     if(CaseRnks[J]<=MinRnk) Minn <- J
    }
   CaseRnks <- sort(CaseRnks)
   LoEE <- CaseRnks[1] - CaseRnks[2]
   HiEE <- CaseRnks[Rnkcols] - CaseRnks[Rnkcols-1]
   for(J in 1:Rnkcols)
    {K <- J + 1
     XtrmXtnt[I,K] <- 0
    }
   if(LoEE<0) XtrmXtnt[I,Minn+1] <- LoEE
   if(HiEE>0) XtrmXtnt[I,Maxx+1] <- HiEE
  }
 XtrmXtnt
}
```

Determination of distal data on the data frame of place-rank data for five variates is done as follows, with parallel boxplots shown in Fig. 9.2:

```
@ DistlData5 <- Xtremity(CasPlacRnk5)
@ boxplot(DistlData5[,-1])
@ tail(DistlData5)
    HexID BirdSp MamlSp ElevSD PctFor PctlFPch
206  4310  -11.0      0    0.0      6        0
207  4311    0.0    -34    0.0      4        0
208  4312    2.0    -24    0.0      0        0
209  4442    4.5     -3    0.0      0        0
210  4443  -39.5      0    0.0      0       18
211  4444    0.0      0   34.5      0       -1
```

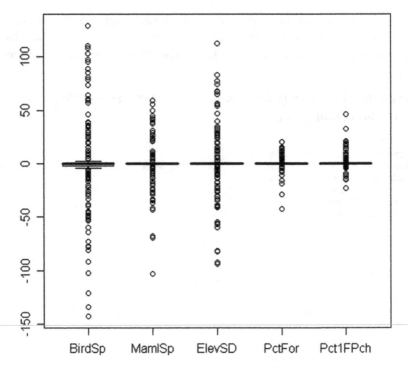

Fig. 9.2 Parallel boxplots of distal data for place ranks of five variates

The hexagons with pronounced extents due to forest variates are found by labeling a plot of Pct1FPch versus PctFor as shown in Fig. 9.3.

```
@ plot(Dist1Data5[,5],Dist1Data5[,6],xlab="PctFor",ylab="Pct1FPch")
@ identify(Dist1Data5[,5],Dist1Data5[,6])
```

The more pronounced extremities in Fig. 9.3 are identified as follows.

```
@ CasPlacRnk5[c(1,77,111,125,27,140),]
    HexID BirdSp MamlSp ElevSD PctFor Pct1FPch
1    1714  211.0  210.5  211.0  193.0    170.0
77   2771   25.0   91.0   78.5  170.5    150.5
111  3144    1.5    8.5   51.5  130.5    163.0
125  3273   11.5   63.0    4.0  111.0    157.0
27   2178  188.5  197.5  179.0  147.0    176.0
140  3519  199.5  112.0  103.5   61.0    121.0
```

Of these, hexagons 2771, 3144, and 3273 stand out as having ranks of forest variates that are much poorer than the ranks of the other three variates. These hexagons are more favorable with respect to vertebrate biodiversity than would be

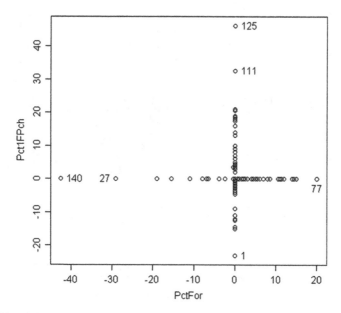

Fig. 9.3 Plot of distal data for Pct1FPch versus distal data for PctFor

expected in view of their lesser forest cover. Therefore, these would be candidates for further investigation in order to understand what leads to these favorable features of vertebrate diversity in the absence of strong forest cover. Selective reforestation might also be pursued to augment this aspect in these areas.

It is also of interest to obtain a cross-plot of distal data for the vertebrate variates as shown in Fig. 9.4.

```
@ plot(DistlData5[,2],DistlData5[,3],xlab="Birds",ylab="Mammals")
@ identify(DistlData5[,2],DistlData5[,3])
```

The first notable feature in the plot of Fig. 9.4 is that the distal departures for birds have a range that is larger than that for the mammals. Distal departures on the low (better) side for mammals are listed as follows. Interestingly, it is only in regard to mammals that these areas have some standing. All other variates have rather inferior ranks. Thus, these are areas in which attention would be on retaining the status for mammals.

```
@ CasPlacRnk5[c(135,146,156),]
    HexID BirdSp MamlSp ElevSD PctFor Pct1FPch
135  3398    166   34.5  137.5    151      159
146  3525    154   63.0  132.5    173      189
156  3653    159   91.0  158.5    186      175
```

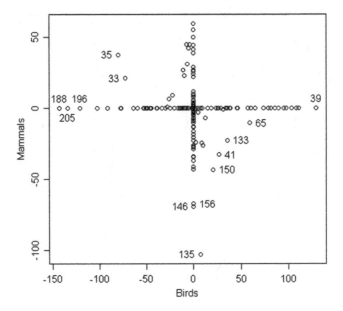

Fig. 9.4 Plot of distal data for mammals versus distal data for birds

Note also that the like-signed quadrants (both negative or both positive) are empty. This is an intrinsic structural feature of the plot since two variates cannot be at the same extremity of the same case. The other two quadrants in Fig. 9.3 were also essentially empty due to the strong correlation between the two variates.

Notably strong status for birds relative to mammals is seen in hexagons 4045, 4309, and 4175. Since all other variates have rather poor placement, retention of bird status would be a focus in these areas.

```
@ CasPlacRnk5[c(188,205,196),]
    HexID BirdSp MamlSp ElevSD PctFor Pct1FPch
188  4045    6.5  149.0  204.0    198      199
205  4309    4.5  138.5  185.5    174      173
196  4175    6.5  127.5  168.0    162      161
```

Disparities in the upper-left quadrant favoring birds are noted for hexagons 2293 and 2291.

```
@ CasPlacRnk5[c(35,33),]
   HexID BirdSp MamlSp ElevSD PctFor Pct1FPch
35  2293   45.0  197.5  125.5  154.0      160
33  2291    1.5  127.5   74.5  106.5       99
```

Hexagons 3529, 2406, 3396, and 2648 form an "arc" of disparities favoring mammals relative to birds in the lower-right quadrant.

```
@ CasPlacRnk5[c(150,41,133,65),]
     HexID BirdSp MamlSp ElevSD PctFor Pct1FPch
150   3529   76.0    1.5   55.5   48.0    45.0
41    2406  116.5   34.5   67.5   89.5    76.5
133   3396  159.0   63.0   86.0  123.5   114.0
65    2648   76.0    4.5   17.0   15.0    15.0
```

Indicator Interaction and Median (Mis)Matching

Much of Part I was devoted to relationships among indicators, all of which are relevant here. If the variates are serving as joint indicators of status under a circumstance, then the indicators should have some commonality of context but not high redundancy. Redundancy entails implicit weighting, whereas there is greater transparency in making any weighting explicit. However, it is counterproductive to include highly discordant indicators, since they speak to a different circumstance and confound analysis of a current focal context.

Since we are dealing here with indicators quantified only as ranks, all other distributional differences have been removed. The simplest investigation of interactions comes in pair plots of the ranked indicators as in Fig. 9.5.

```
@ pairs(CasPlacRnk5[,-1])
```

A basic statistical approach is to examine correlations among the rankings of the indicators, which is the Spearman rank correlation coefficient that was computed earlier. When working directly with ranks, the usual (Pearson) correlation coefficient is equivalent to Spearman correlation for the raw data, except for possible slight perturbation from different methods of handling tied ranks.

```
@ cor(CasPlacRnk5[,-1])
             BirdSp     MamlSp     ElevSD     PctFor   Pct1FPch
BirdSp    1.0000000  0.5790877  0.4339592  0.1648744  0.1638723
MamlSp    0.5790877  1.0000000  0.6298376  0.4926405  0.4640142
ElevSD    0.4339592  0.6298376  1.0000000  0.4495578  0.4245905
PctFor    0.1648744  0.4926405  0.4495578  1.0000000  0.9826981
Pct1FPch  0.1638723  0.4640142  0.4245905  0.9826981  1.0000000
```

Correlations are moderate, except for a high correlation between the two forest variates and low correlation between BirdSp and the two forest variates. The very high correlation between the two forest variates implies redundancy and attendant implicit weighting. Therefore, it would be in order to drop the last variate and work with only the remaining four. Before doing so, however, it would be prudent to check on at least those cases that lie farthest from the general trend of these two variates.

It should be noted that redundancy does not impair these comparative rating regimes for ascribing advantage, except with regard to extremities of distal data.

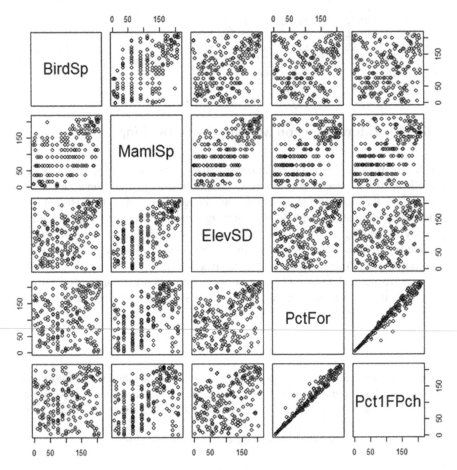

Fig. 9.5 Pairs plot of rank data for all hexagons on five indicators

In dropping indicators, it also must be kept in mind that interactions could be different if a different set of cases were to be studied. Since the BirdSp indicator does show moderate rank correlation with MamlSp and ElevSD, it is not idiosyncratic in its overall behavior. Notably, Fig. 9.5 shows that the low association between BirdSp and forest variates is not just due to a specific suite of inconsistent cases.

We can also borrow from the ideas of cross-validation and residuals to explore how well or poorly the rank of each indicator corresponds with the median rank of the other indicators. The MdnMsMch Function 9.2 serves to determine the mismatches in this regard. The median mismatches can then be presented in pair plots in the manner of Fig. 9.6.

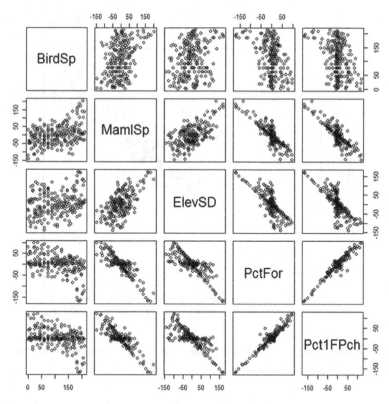

Fig. 9.6 Pair plots for median mismatches that arise in predicting the rank of each metric from the median rank of the other metrics

Function 9.2: MdnMsMch Function for Determining Difference between Indicator Rank and Median of Ranks for other Indicators

```
MdnMsMch <- function(RankData)
# RankData is a data frame of place ranks as produced by PlacRank
        function.
# MisMtchs is a data frame of mismatches with median rank of other
        indicators.
{RnkCols <- length(RankData)
 Rnkcols <- RnkCols - 1
 Cases <- length(RankData[,1])
 RnkData <- RankData
 for(I in 1:Cases)
  {CaseRnks <- rep(0,Rnkcols)
   for(J in 1:Rnkcols)
    {K <- J + 1
     CaseRnks[J] <- RankData[I,K]
    }
   for(J in 1:Rnkcols)
    {K <- J + 1
     Medn <- median(CaseRnks[-J])
     MisMtch <- CaseRnks[J] - Medn
     RnkData[I,K] <- MisMtch
    }
  }
 RnkData
}
```

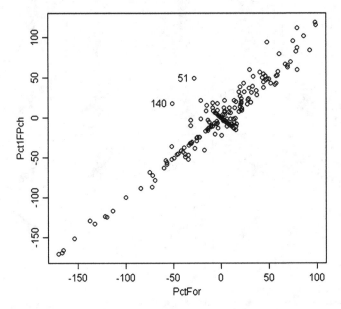

Fig. 9.7 Median mismatches for percent in one forest patch (*Y*-axis) versus percent forest (*X*-axis)

Applying the MdnMsMch function gives the following:

```
@ MisMatch <- MdnMsMch(CasPlacRnk5[,-1])
@ head(MisMatch)
  BirdSp MamlSp ElevSD PctFor Pct1FPch
1  211.0   17.5   18.0  -17.5    -40.5
2  210.0  136.0  121.5 -121.5   -123.5
3  159.0   40.0   34.5  -34.5    -52.5
4  202.5    8.5    6.0   -6.0    -21.0
5  204.0  203.0  132.5 -132.5   -132.5
6  148.0   80.5   72.5  -72.5    -87.0
@ pairs(MisMatch)
```

The pair plots of median mismatches in Fig. 9.6 again show general relationships among the indicators, but also provide better perspective on which cases exhibit peculiarities of interactions among indicators, such as between forest and topography. For example, plotting ranks of the percent in one forest patch on the *Y*-axis against percent forest on the *X*-axis (Fig. 9.7) draws attention to hexagons 2524 and 3519 as being particularly fragmented since their ranks on PctFor are relatively favorable but considerably less soon Pct1FPch. This reflects substantial forest cover occurring in a patchy pattern.

```
@ plot(MisMatch[,4],MisMatch[,5],xlab="PctFor",ylab="Pct1FPch")
@ identify(MisMatch[,4],MisMatch[,5])
[1]  51 140
@ CasPlacRnk5[c(51,140),]
     HexID BirdSp MamlSp ElevSD PctFor Pct1FPch
51    2524  194.5     63    2.0     35       84
140   3519  199.5    112  103.5     61      121
```

Conditional Complement

Situations may also arise in which prioritization is being conducted in a progressive manner such that the highest priority cases have been determined and it is further desired to identify additional cases which would best complement the current ones by compensating for any shortcomings. This can be addressed by constructing a composite case in which each indicator variate is given the minimum (place) rank that any of the current selections have for that variate. Alterations are then made in the (place) rank values for the remaining candidates by assigning that of the composite if it is under (less than) the actual rank. Advantage then accrues to a candidate only if it has one or more ranks that are under those of the composite, i.e., better than any among the current selections. This strategy underscores the flexibility of the current comparative approach and its application is included in the next chapter.

Reference

Newlin J, Bhat K (2007) Identification and prioritization of stream channel maintenance needs at bridge crossings. In: Proceedings of the international bridge conference, IBC 07-18, Pittsburgh, PA

Chapter 10
Landscape Linkage for Prioritizing Proximate Patches

From among the protocols of the previous chapters, we first carry forward "salient scaling" as ranked ORDITs from applying product-order protocols to place-ranked criteria. This chapter extends the foregoing by incorporating spatial linkage criteria (Bivand et al. 2008) with the salient scaling to construct a contiguous area on the landscape from component cells (hexagons) that might serve the interests of conservation. For present purposes, we focus attention on hexagons in the Ridge and Valley Region of Pennsylvania (Fig. 10.1).

The first four variates will again serve as favorable conservation criteria, but the fifth variate (Pct1FPch) will be omitted since the previous chapter showed a high degree of redundancy with PctFor which is the fourth variate. These indicators are shown in Table 10.1. The last variate for each hexagon is percentage in one single contiguous open (nonforested) patch (Pct1OPch), which was not previously used as an indicator. This time, however, we will view this variate as being counter-indicative for conservation, and this will provide criteria for the quality of linkage between adjacent hexagons. A separate data file (RVpairs.txt) of neighbor relations between hexagons that also contains the open-patch percentage data for both members of an adjacent pair is prepared as shown in Table 10.2, where hexagons are called zones and Pct1OPch is referred to as "Open". Zone (hexagon) ID numbers are critical to the current analysis, and must appear in first column and first two columns of these data files, respectively.

Functions again play a central role in this scenario. All computations for salient scaling are folded into one function called Salient which takes a frame of place-rank data and a vector of zone ID numbers as its inputs (Function 10.1). This function orders zones (hexagons) according to salient scaling from best to worst.

W.L. Myers and G.P. Patil, *Multivariate Methods of Representing Relations in R for Prioritization Purposes*, Environmental and Ecological Statistics 6, DOI 10.1007/978-1-4614-3122-0_10, © Springer Science+Business Media, LLC 2012

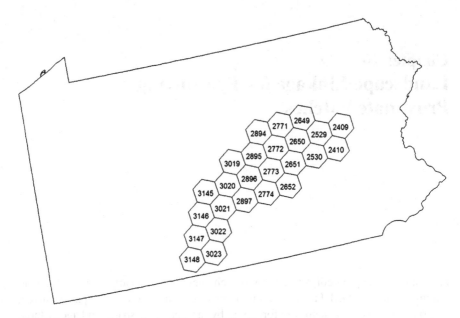

Fig. 10.1 Hexagonal zones in the Ridge and Valley Region

Table 10.1 Conservation characteristics for hexagonal cells in the Ridge and Valley Region of Pennsylvania

ZoneNum	BirdSp	MamlSp	TopoVarI	PctForst
2409	130	45	89	80.8
2410	128	43	105	85.4
2529	133	45	103	74.3
2530	123	45	83	82.5
2649	127	47	65	66.0
2650	120	46	56	69.8
2651	121	46	62	62.5
2652	129	45	70	80.1
2771	135	47	81	48.9
2772	130	46	54	47.5
2773	122	46	101	76.6
2774	126	46	80	77.1
2894	126	47	114	89.4
2895	135	47	130	84.7
2896	123	49	114	75.4
2897	129	48	114	83.2
3019	133	53	102	59.3
3020	136	51	117	68.7
3021	122	46	110	89.8
3022	128	47	123	87.0
3023	118	46	110	74.4
3145	131	50	94	67.4
3146	128	48	103	68.8
3147	129	48	94	69.7
3148	120	47	92	78.1

Table 10.2 Neighbor relations for ridge and valley hexagonal zones with open-patch percentages

ZoneA	ZoneB	OpenA	OpenB
2409	2410	11.2	4.0
2409	2529	11.2	7.6
2410	2530	4.0	9.4
2529	2649	7.6	8.5
2529	2650	7.6	5.5
2529	2530	7.6	9.4
2529	2410	7.6	4.0
2530	2651	9.4	11.1
2649	2771	8.5	30.4
2649	2650	8.5	5.5
2771	2894	30.4	4.5
2771	2772	30.4	22.3
2771	2650	30.4	5.5
2650	2772	5.5	22.3
2650	2651	5.5	11.1
2650	2530	5.5	9.4
2651	2773	11.1	6.7
2651	2652	11.1	5.1
2652	2774	5.1	10.3
2894	2895	4.5	6.3
2894	2772	4.5	22.3
2772	2895	22.3	6.3
2772	2773	22.3	6.7
2772	2651	22.3	11.1
2895	3019	6.3	23.4
2895	2896	6.3	6.6
2895	2773	6.3	6.7
2773	2896	6.7	6.6
2773	2774	6.7	10.3
2773	2652	6.7	5.1
2774	2897	10.3	8.8
3019	3020	23.4	16.7
3019	2896	23.4	6.6
2896	3020	6.6	16.7
2896	2897	6.6	8.8
2896	2774	6.6	10.3
2897	3021	8.8	2.0
3020	3145	16.7	11.1
3020	3021	16.7	2.0
3020	2897	16.7	8.8
3145	3146	11.1	23.1
3145	3021	11.1	2.0
3021	3146	2.0	23.1
3021	3022	2.0	4.4
3146	3147	23.1	13.9
3146	3022	23.1	4.4
3147	3148	13.9	7.8
3147	3022	13.9	4.4
3147	3023	13.9	5.1
3022	3023	4.4	5.1
3023	3148	5.1	7.8

Function 10.1: Salient Function for Order of Salient Scaling Based on Place-Ranks

```
Salient <- function(Rankings,CaseIDs)
{Ncol <- length(Rankings)
 Ncase <- length(Rankings[,1])
 Status1 <- rep(-1,Ncase)
 Status2 <- Status1
 DD <- Ncase - 1
 for(I in 1:Ncase)
  {Nosub <- 0; Levl <- 0
    for(J in 1:Ncase)
     {if(I<J | I>J)
       {MatchA <- 0; MatchB <- 0; Undom <- 1
        VecA <- Rankings[J,] - Rankings[I,]
        if(max(VecA) > 0) MatchA <- 1
        if(min(VecA) < 0) MatchB <- 1
        if(MatchA==1 & MatchB==0) Nosub <- Nosub + 1
        if(MatchA==0 & MatchB==1) Undom <- 0
        Levl <- Levl + Undom
        }
     }
    Status1[I] <- Nosub
    Status2[I] <- DD - Levl
  }
 AA <- Status1
 SS <- Status2
 Pct <- 100/DD
 AA <- AA * Pct
 AA <- round(AA,digits=2)
 SS <- SS * Pct
 SS <- round(SS,digits=2)
 ccc <- rep(0,Ncase)
 bbb <- ccc
 ORDIT <- ccc
 for(I in 1:Ncase)
  {ccc[I] <- (100 - AA[I]) * 100
    ccc[I] <- round(ccc[I],digits=0)
    if(AA[I] < 100) bbb[I] <- SS[I]/(100 - AA[I])
    if(bbb[I] > 0.999) bbb[I] <- 0.999
    bbb[I] <- round(bbb[I],digits=3)
    ORDIT[I] <- ccc[I] + bbb[I]
  }
 Salnt <- rank(ORDIT)
 Salients <- cbind(CaseIDs,Salnt)
 SalntOrdr <- order(Salnt)
 Salients <- Salients[SalntOrdr,]
 Salients
}
```

The first task is to use the Salient function to determine which one or adjacent ones of the hexagons should serve to anchor the expanding sector as core component(s). The actual choice of which one(s) of the zones to use at each step of the progression is left to the discretion and expertise of the analyst so that the salient scale ratings serve in an advisory capacity. The initial determination for anchor zone(s) is based on the data in Table 10.1 without regard to the data on pairings in Table 10.2. Thereafter, the quality of the linkages between pairs also enters into the considerations. If expert intervention is exercised at any given juncture, the onward trajectory of development still builds objectively upon that expert intervention.

When anchor elements (hexagonal zones) have been chosen, then Function 10.2 named Primary is used to set up the frame onto which other zones will be annexed in subsequent stages. This frame has stage of development in its first column, and zone numbers entering in that stage as its second column. The only input to the primary function is a vector of zone number(s) to serve as the core.

Function 10.2: Primary Function for Setting Up Frame of Zones at Initial Stage

```
Primary <- function(Starting)
{Siz <- length(Starting)
 Stage <- rep(0,Siz)
 Zones <- Starting
 Sector <- cbind(Stage,Zones)
 Sector
}
```

Given the foregoing functions along with the PlacRank function from previous chapters, the initial computations are as follows by which hexagon 2895 is selected as anchor.

```
@ RVhexs <- read.table("RVhexs.txt",header=T)
@ RVpairs <- read.table("RVpairs.txt",header=T)
@ head(RVhexs)
  ZoneNum BirdSp MamlSp TopoVarI PctForst
1    2409    130     45       89     80.8
2    2410    128     43      105     85.4
3    2529    133     45      103     74.3
4    2530    123     45       83     82.5
5    2649    127     47       65     66.0
6    2650    120     46       56     69.8
@ RVhexIDs <- RVhexs[,1]
@ RVhexRank <- PlacRank(RVhexs[,-1])
@ RVhexOrd <- Salient(RVhexRank,RVhexIDs)
```

```
@ head(RVhexOrd)
      CaseIDs Salnt
[1,]     2895      1
[2,]     2897      2
[3,]     3022      3
[4,]     2894      4
[5,]     3020      5
[6,]     3021      6
@ FirstHex <- 2895
@ HexSet <- Primary(FirstHex)
@ HexSet
       Stage Zones
[1,]       0  2895
```

After the anchor is in place, all of the subsequent expansion stages follow a common pattern. First, the bordering zones for the current set must be determined and a corresponding frame of indicators assembled. This is the purpose of the Fringe Function 10.3, which requires the hexagon (zone) data, pairing data, and set of zones as a staging frame. For the current context, hexagons 2894, 2772, 3019, 2896, and 2773 comprise the border. All interior hexagon indicators are labeled simply as "ZoneX".

```
@ Border <- Fringe(RVhexs,RVpairs,HexSet)
@ Border
    ZoneA OpenA OpenB ZoneX ZoneX ZoneX ZoneX
20   2894   4.5   6.3   126    47   114  89.4
22   2772  22.3   6.3   130    46    54  47.5
25   3019   6.3  23.4   133    53   102  59.3
26   2896   6.3   6.6   123    49   114  75.4
27   2773   6.3   6.7   122    46   101  76.6
```

The border frame is then split into zone IDs and place-ranked indicators as follows.

```
@ BorderIDs <- Border[,1]
@ BorderRnks <- PlacRank(Border[,-1])
```

However, the first two "open" features are counter-indicative, and must undergo regular ranking instead of place ranking.

```
@ BorderRnks[,1] <- rank(Border[,2])
@ BorderRnks[,2] <- rank(Border[,3])
```

Function 10.3: Fringe Function for Bordering Zones

```
Fringe <- function(ZoneData,ZoneEdge,ZoneSet)
{ZoneEdg <- ZoneEdge
 EdgItems <- length(ZoneEdg[,1])
 ZonSets <- length(ZoneSet[,1])
 ZonVars <- length(ZoneData) - 1
 Zons <- length(ZoneData[,1])
 for(I in 1:EdgItems)
  {Ia <- 0; Ib <- 0
   EdgA <- ZoneEdg[I,1]; EdgB <- ZoneEdg[I,2]
   for(J in 1:ZonSets)
    {if(EdgA==ZoneSet[J,2]) Ia <- 1
     if(EdgB==ZoneSet[J,2]) Ib <- 1
    }
   if(Ia==1 & Ib==0) ZoneEdg[I,1] <- EdgB
   if(Ia==1 & Ib==1) ZoneEdg[I,1] <- 0
   if(Ia==0 & Ib==0) ZoneEdg[I,1] <- 0
  }
 ZoneEdg <- ZoneEdg[,-2]
 Chk <- length(ZoneEdg)
 Chek <- ZoneEdg[,1]
 ZoneEdg <- ZoneEdg[Chek>0,]
 Chek <- length(ZoneEdg[,1])
 ZoneX <- rep(0,Chek)
 for(I in 1:ZonVars) ZoneEdg <- cbind(ZoneEdg,ZoneX)
 Border <- ZoneEdg
 for(I in 1:Chek)
  {for(J in 1:Zons)
    {if(Border[I,1]==ZoneData[J,1])
      {for(K in 1:ZonVars)
        {Ia <- K + 1; Ib <- Chk + K
         Border[I,Ib] <- ZoneData[J,Ia]
        }
      }
    }
  }
 Border
}
```

The border IDs and border ranks can now be submitted for salient scale rating, which poses hexagon 2894 as the candidate to be annexed for expansion.

```
@ BorderOrd <- Salient(BorderRnks,BorderIDs)
@ BorderOrd
     CaseIDs Salnt
[1,]    2894     1
[2,]    2772     3
[3,]    3019     3
[4,]    2896     3
[5,]    2773     5
```

The annexation is accomplished with the Annex Function 10.4, which takes the current set of zones (HexSet) and expansion zones as inputs.

Function 10.4: Annex Function for Incorporating Zones of the Current Expansion

```
Annex <- function(InPlace,AddOns)
{OldStage <- InPlace[,1]
 OldZones <- InPlace[,2]
 NuSiz <- length(OldZones) + length(AddOns)
 Zones <- rep(0,NuSiz)
 NexStag <- max(OldStage) + 1
 Stage <- rep(NexStag,NuSiz)
 OldSiz <- length(OldZones)
 for(I in 1:OldSiz)
  {Stage[I] <- OldStage[I]
   Zones[I] <- OldZones[I]
  }
 NuOne <- OldSiz + 1
 J <- 0
 for(I in NuOne:NuSiz)
  {J <- J + 1
   Zones[I] <- AddOns[J]
  }
 Sector <- cbind(Stage,Zones)
 Sector
}

@ Xpand <- 2894
@ HexSet <- Annex(HexSet,Xpand)
@ HexSet
     Stage Zones
[1,]     0  2895
[2,]     1  2894
```

   This completes one expansion cycle. The steps for subsequent expansion cycles are the same, and are given together with annotation but without other commentary in the following. Note that border zone 2772 shows up twice. This is because that zone borders two (both) of the current hexagons, and linkage criteria can be different for the two couplings; however, it should only be annexed once. Since all of the border zones have the same salient score, the entire border is annexed at this stage.

```
@ #Determine Border
@ Border <- Fringe(RVhexs,RVpairs,HexSet)
@ Border
   ZoneA OpenA OpenB ZoneX ZoneX ZoneX ZoneX
11  2771  30.4   4.5   135    47    81  48.9
21  2772   4.5  22.3   130    46    54  47.5
22  2772  22.3   6.3   130    46    54  47.5
25  3019   6.3  23.4   133    53   102  59.3
26  2896   6.3   6.6   123    49   114  75.4
27  2773   6.3   6.7   122    46   101  76.6
@ #Split Border frame
@ BorderIDs <- Border[,1]
@ BorderRnks <- PlacRank(Border[,-1])
@ #Rank two counter-indicators
@ BorderRnks[,1] <- rank(Border[,2])
@ BorderRnks[,2] <- rank(Border[,3])
@ #Ordination of Border zones by salient scaling
@ BorderOrd <- Salient(BorderRnks,BorderIDs)
@ BorderOrd
       CaseIDs Salnt
[1,]    2771    3.5
[2,]    2772    3.5
[3,]    2772    3.5
[4,]    3019    3.5
[5,]    2896    3.5
[6,]    2773    3.5
@ #Annexation
@ Xpand <- BorderOrd[-2,1]
@ HexSet <- Annex(HexSet,Xpand)
@ HexSet
       Stage Zones
[1,]     0   2895
[2,]     1   2894
[3,]     2   2771
[4,]     2   2772
[5,]     2   3019
[6,]     2   2896
[7,]     2   2773
```

Decisions regarding when to halt the expansion can be made according to several considerations, including the desired size of the sector and the collective salient scale ratings as obtained in the initial stage. The current context can be viewed in the larger sense of extracting a priority portion of a more general network. In this larger sense, the zones are nodes in the network and the (border) pairings are the links in the network, with prioritization being done jointly on properties of the nodes and links. Thus, this approach has considerable generality.

Contiguous Complement

We now revisit the foregoing scenario with different data for the same spatial units in order to add a second perspective. This time the main indicators are species richness of four vertebrate taxa: birds, mammals, herpetiles (snakes, lizards, amphibians), and fish as given in Table 10.3. The spatial linkage criterion is percent forest (Table 10.4), taken as a positive indicator. The focus is on choosing a contiguous

Table 10.3 Species richness of four vertebrate taxa for hexagonal cells in the Ridge and Valley Region of Pennsylvania

ZoneNum	BirdSp	MamlSp	HerpSp	FishSp
2409	130	45	16	31
2410	128	43	18	29
2529	133	45	21	32
2530	123	45	19	30
2649	127	47	23	32
2650	120	46	26	35
2651	121	46	20	38
2652	129	45	33	44
2771	135	47	30	36
2772	130	46	33	42
2773	122	46	23	37
2774	126	46	33	43
2894	126	47	25	31
2895	135	47	37	32
2896	123	49	26	38
2897	129	48	30	39
3019	133	53	31	42
3020	136	51	33	33
3021	122	46	31	41
3022	128	47	29	39
3023	118	46	30	33
3145	131	50	34	37
3146	128	48	34	39
3147	129	48	37	36
3148	120	47	27	33

Table 10.4 Neighbor relations for ridge and valley hexagonal zones with forest cover percentages

ZoneA	ZoneB	PctForA	PctForB
2409	2410	80.8	85.4
2409	2529	80.8	74.3
2410	2530	85.4	82.5
2529	2649	74.3	66.0
2529	2650	74.3	69.8
2529	2530	74.3	82.5
2529	2410	74.3	85.4
2530	2651	82.5	62.5
2649	2771	66.0	48.9
2649	2650	66.0	69.8
2771	2894	48.9	89.4
2771	2772	48.9	47.5
2771	2650	48.9	69.8
2650	2772	69.8	47.5
2650	2651	69.8	62.5
2650	2530	69.8	82.5
2651	2773	62.5	76.6
2651	2652	62.5	80.1
2652	2774	80.1	77.1
2894	2895	89.4	84.7
2894	2772	89.4	47.5
2772	2895	47.5	84.7
2772	2773	47.5	76.6
2772	2651	47.5	62.5
2895	3019	84.7	59.3
2895	2896	84.7	75.4
2895	2773	84.7	76.6
2773	2896	76.6	75.4
2773	2774	76.6	77.1
2773	2652	76.6	80.1
2774	2897	77.1	83.2
3019	3020	59.3	68.7
3019	2896	59.3	75.4
2896	3020	75.4	68.7
2896	2897	75.4	83.2
2896	2774	75.4	77.1
2897	3021	83.2	89.8
3020	3145	68.7	67.4
3020	3021	68.7	89.8
3020	2897	68.7	83.2
3145	3146	67.4	68.8
3145	3021	67.4	89.8
3021	3146	89.8	68.8
3021	3022	89.8	87.0
3146	3147	68.8	69.7
3146	3022	68.8	87.0
3147	3148	69.7	78.1
3147	3022	69.7	87.0
3147	3023	69.7	74.4
3022	3023	87.0	74.4
3023	3148	74.4	78.1

area of high biodiversity. However, it is not necessarily expected to be such that all kinds of biodiversity are high in the same cell. For example, herps and fish tend to be more in lowland and river settings with many birds favoring extensive upland forest settings. Thus, each cycle of expansion will entail two perspectives on precedence. One is the usual perspective of overall quality. The second perspective considers the candidates that best complement current choices by compensating for deficiencies whereby one or more of the taxa are not well represented among the previous choices.

We begin by obtaining an anchor unit as before, but with appropriate changes in file names.

```
@ RVhexsp <- read.table("RVsprich.txt",header=T)
@ RVpairsp <- read.table("RVfpairs.txt",header=T)
@ head(RVhexsp)
  ZoneNum BirdSp MamlSp HerpSp FishSp
1    2409    130     45     16     31
2    2410    128     43     18     29
3    2529    133     45     21     32
4    2530    123     45     19     30
5    2649    127     47     23     32
6    2650    120     46     26     35
@ RVhexID <- RVhexsp[,1]
@ RVhexRnk <- PlacRank(RVhexsp[,-1])
@ RVhexOrds <- Salient(RVhexRnk,RVhexID)
@ head(RVhexOrds)
      CaseIDs Salnt
[1,]     3019   1.0
[2,]     3146   2.0
[3,]     2897   3.0
[4,]     2771   4.5
[5,]     3145   4.5
[6,]     2772   6.5
@ FrstHex <- 3019
@ HexSetsp <- Primary(FrstHex)
@ HexSetsp
      Stage Zones
[1,]      0  3019
```

The only commonality with the previous scenario among the top three candidates is hexagon 2897, which was previously second and is now third. Hexagon 3019 is superior in all four taxa to 2897, and superior to 2895 in all taxa except for herps. Hexagon 3019 is thus chosen as the anchor for the biodiversity set.

The first perspective on an expansion again follows the previous pattern starting with the Fringe function and then place ranking. This time the linkage criteria (percent forest) are positively indicative, so reranking does not occur and the place ranks can be submitted directly to the Salient function.

```
@ Bordrsp <- Fringe(RVhexsp,RVpairsp,HexSetsp)
@ Bordrsp
   ZoneA PctForA PctForB ZoneX ZoneX ZoneX ZoneX
25  2895    84.7    59.3   135    47    37    32
32  3020    59.3    68.7   136    51    33    33
33  2896    59.3    75.4   123    49    26    38
@ BordrID <- Bordrsp[,1]
@ BordrRnks <- PlacRank(Bordrsp[,-1])
@ BordrOrd <- Salient(BordrRnks,BordrID)
@ BordrOrd
       CaseIDs Salnt
[1,]     2895      2
[2,]     3020      2
[3,]     2896      2
```

All three border hexagons are recommended for expansion from this first perspective. The second perspective is complementary to the prior selection of 3019 as anchor (regardless of forest linkage conditions) in terms of biodiversity ratings. As mentioned in the previous chapter, the complementary perspective can be approached by constructing a composite case in which each indicator variate is given the minimum (place) rank that any of the current selections have for that variate. Alterations are then made in the (place) rank values for the remaining candidates by assigning that of the composite if it is under (less than) the actual rank. Advantage will then accrue to a candidate only if it has one or more ranks that are under those of the composite, i.e., better than any among the current selections. This approach is enabled for the present setting by the Complmnt Function 10.5. This function takes four inputs which are respectively a vector containing the IDs of the elements (cases) previously chosen, a vector containing the IDs of the elements currently eligible to be chosen, a vector containing the IDs for all elements, and a data frame containing place ranks for all elements in the same order as the IDs. For the current situation, only the border elements (hexagonal cells) are eligible to be chosen. The Complmnt function returns a data frame of complementary ratings, which should be submitted directly to the Salient function.

```
@ RVcmplmnt <- Complmnt(HexSetsp[,2],BordrID,RVhexID,RVhexRnk)
@ RVcmplmnt
  BirdSp MamlSp HerpSp FishSp
1    2.5      1    1.5    3.5
2    4.5      1    9.5    3.5
3    1.0      1    6.5    3.5
@ CmplmntOrd <- Salient(RVcmplmnt,BordrID)
@ CmplmntOrd
       CaseIDs Salnt
[1,]     2895    1.5
[2,]     2896    1.5
[3,]     3020    3.0
```

Function 10.5: Complmnt Function for Assigning Complementary Ratings in Progressive Expansion of Selections

Inputs are respectively a vector containing the IDs of the elements (cases) previously chosen, a vector containing the IDs of the elements currently eligible to be chosen, a vector containing the IDs for all elements, and a data frame containing place ranks for all elements in the same order as the IDs.

```
Complmnt <- function(PriorIDs,ElgblIDs,AllIDs,AllRanks)
{Nratings <- length(AllRanks)
 Nrated <- length(AllIDs)
 Nprior <- length(PriorIDs)
 Nelgbl <- length(ElgblIDs)
 Composit <- rep(0,Nratings)
 Bgin <- 0
 #Construct composite
 for(I in 1:Nrated)
  {for(J in 1:Nprior)
    {if(PriorIDs[J]==AllIDs[I])
      {if(Bgin==0)
        {for(K in 1:Nratings) Composit[K] <- AllRanks[I,K]
          Bgin <- 1
         }
       for(K in 1:Nratings)
        if(AllRanks[I,K]<Composit[K]) Composit[K] <- AllRanks[I,K]
      }
    }
  }
 #Construct complements
 RelRanks <- AllRanks[1:Nelgbl,]
 M <- 1
 for(I in 1:Nrated)
  {for(J in 1:Nelgbl)
    {if(AllIDs[I]==ElgblIDs[J])
      {for(K in 1:Nratings) RelRanks[M,K] <- AllRanks[I,K]
       M <- M + 1
      }
    }
  }
 for(I in 1:Nelgbl)
  {for(J in 1:Nratings)
   if(Composit[J]<RelRanks[I,J]) RelRanks[I,J] <- Composit[J]
  }
 RelRanks
}
```

From the complementary perspective, hexagon 2895 is tied with 2896 and 3020 has less precedence. Therefore, 2895 and 2896 should both be annexed in this first cycle of expansion.

```
@ Xpands <- c(2895,2896)
@ HexSetsp <- Annex(HexSetsp,Xpands)
@ HexSetsp
      Stage Zones
[1,]      0  3019
[2,]      1  2895
[3,]      1  2896
```

Subsequent cycles of expansion transpire in like manner with consideration of both perspectives. For the first perspective this is again as follows, highlighting hexagons 2773 and 3020.

```
@ Bordrsp <- Fringe(RVhexsp,RVpairsp,HexSetsp)
@ Bordrsp
   ZoneA PctForA PctForB ZoneX ZoneX ZoneX ZoneX
20  2894    89.4    84.7   126    47    25    31
22  2772    47.5    84.7   130    46    33    42
27  2773    84.7    76.6   122    46    23    37
28  2773    76.6    75.4   122    46    23    37
32  3020    59.3    68.7   136    51    33    33
34  3020    75.4    68.7   136    51    33    33
35  2897    75.4    83.2   129    48    30    39
36  2774    75.4    77.1   126    46    33    43
@ BordrID <- Bordrsp[,1]
@ BordrRnks <- PlacRank(Bordrsp[,-1])
@ BordrOrd <- Salient(BordrRnks,BordrID)
@ BordrOrd
      CaseIDs Salnt
[1,]     2773   1.5
[2,]     3020   1.5
[3,]     2894   4.5
[4,]     2772   4.5
[5,]     2897   4.5
[6,]     2774   4.5
[7,]     2773   7.5
[8,]     3020   7.5
```

The complementary perspective is then obtained, with 2773, 2774, and 2897 all being tied.

```
@ RVcmplmnt <- Complmnt(HexSetsp[,2],BordrID,RVhexID,RVhexRnk)
@ RVcmplmnt
  BirdSp MamlSp HerpSp FishSp
1   2.5       1    1.5    3.5
2   2.5       1    1.5    3.5
3   2.5       1    1.5    3.5
4   2.5       1    1.5    2.0
5   2.5       1    1.5    3.5
6   2.5       1    1.5    3.5
7   1.0       1    1.5    3.5
8   1.0       1    1.5    3.5
@ CmplmntOrd <- Salient(RVcmplmnt,BordrID)
```

```
@ CmplmntOrd
       CaseIDs Salnt
[1,]      2773     2
[2,]      2897     2
[3,]      2774     2
[4,]      2894     6
[5,]      2772     6
[6,]      2773     6
[7,]      3020     6
[8,]      3020     6
```

Both perspectives have consensus on 2773 with both 2774 and 2897 being more complementary than 3020. Therefore, these three are annexed.

```
@ Xpands <- c(2773,2774,2897)
@ HexSetsp <- Annex(HexSetsp,Xpands)
@ HexSetsp
     Stage Zones
[1,]     0  3019
[2,]     1  2895
[3,]     1  2896
[4,]     2  2773
[5,]     2  2774
[6,]     2  2897
```

It thus becomes evident that the complementary perspective is not necessarily the same as choosing units that are next best in an overall sense.

Reference

Bivand R, Pebesma E, Gomez-Rubio V (2008) Applied spatial data analysis with R. Springer, New York

Chapter 11
Constellations of Criteria

It is not uncommon for different kinds of considerations to enter into a prioritization context. Each consideration can have a constellation of indicators, and these constellations may be complementary or conflicting. Data on such an Italian context come from Angelo Pecci (personal communication) working with Prof. Orazio Rossi at University of Parma in relation to Italian Map of Nature on data from ISPRA and Ministry of Environment of Italy (Rossi et al. 2008). Basic ecological assessment is conducted at the level of a contiguous tract (ecotope) of a designated type. One constellation of indicators speaks to ecological value, and another constellation of indicators speaks to ecological sensitivity (to disruptions). Compilations have been done for ecological value and sensitivity over civil divisions called communes. Each commune thus has a suite (constellation) of indicators for ecological value and another for ecological sensitivity. Additionally, each commune has a constellation of indicators that speaks to human pressure on the natural elements. One situation of interest is to determine communes where there is high ecological value that also has high sensitivity in company with high human pressure. Such communes would be candidates for what might be called conservation crisis intervention through special funding programs. The data covers 108 communes, for which we are not presently concerned with their specific identity or location. Only what emerges analytically from the data is given here so that the data and identities remain anonymous.

One of the interesting aspects of this particular context is that ecological value and ecological sensitivity can be seen as having some complementary sense. However, human pressure generally tends to be the bane of the ecological aspects, and thus primarily conflicting with regard to indications. However, there can be situations were ecological elements are imbedded in zones that otherwise have high human pressure. Such imbedding can be as parks, preserves, sanctuaries, or local landscapes that have a topographic character that is more conducive to tourism than to industrial, commercial, or residential development.

W.L. Myers and G.P. Patil, *Multivariate Methods of Representing Relations in R for Prioritization Purposes*, Environmental and Ecological Statistics 6, DOI 10.1007/978-1-4614-3122-0_11, © Springer Science+Business Media, LLC 2012

Data Format

These data reside in Microsoft Excel spreadsheets, which is a frequent format that has not been addressed in any of what has been presented. **R** does have a document that speaks to "**R** Data Import/Export". With respect to Excel spreadsheets, this document recommends saving the spreadsheet as a tab-delimited text file. The delimited file can then be read into **R** with the `read.delim()` command. For example, the ecological value spreadsheet could be saved as EVdelim.txt and then read into **R** as: `EV <- read.delim("EVdelim.txt",header=T)`

This approach has been used in the present circumstance to access the data in **R**. Having accessed a particular spreadsheet in **R**, the `write.table()` command was then used to write a file that can be read subsequently with the usual `read.table()` command.

Ecological Value Indicators

Nine indicators of ecological value were provided, all of which were viewed as being positively indicative. For present purposes, a decision has been made here to drop two of these due to preponderance of zeros. One of these concerned percent in protected areas, and the other concerned involvement in conservation areas. The remaining seven were place-ranked, with the first entry in the data frame of place ranks being the identification number for the commune. The data frame of place ranks was then written (with `write.table`) to a file having EcoValuR.txt as its name. From this, a `pairs()` plot of the ranks was prepared as follows (Fig. 11.1).

```
@ EcoValuR <- read.table("EcoValuR.txt",header=T)
@ pairs(EcoValuR[,-1])
```

It can be seen that several of the indicators are strongly correlated, and the V_ RARITY indicator has special influence by virtue of its partial stratifying effect.

The correlation matrix for the ranked ecological value data (excluding IDs) is obtained as follows.

```
@ cor(EcoValuR[,-1])
                VERT_RICH     H_RARITY      V_RARITY SOIL_ROUGH     VR_SUIT
VERT_RICH     1.000000000    0.5326417   0.456263638  0.8401021   0.9384305
H_RARITY      0.532641678    1.0000000   0.247182765  0.3722890   0.5430178
V_RARITY      0.456263638    0.2471828   1.000000000  0.4458025   0.2705229
SOIL_ROUGH    0.840102127    0.3722890   0.445802469  1.0000000   0.8331114
VR_SUIT       0.938430503    0.5430178   0.270522940  0.8331114   1.0000000
NDVI          0.964386341    0.5205508   0.471506735  0.8198310   0.8988963
SIZE_HA      -0.002996194   -0.1029200  -0.006395494  0.3799450   0.1016612
                    NDVI       SIZE_HA
VERT_RICH     0.96438634  -0.002996194
H_RARITY      0.52055085  -0.102920021
V_RARITY      0.47150673  -0.006395494
SOIL_ROUGH    0.81983104   0.379945030
VR_SUIT       0.89889631   0.101661248
NDVI          1.00000000  -0.015647887
SIZE_HA      -0.01564789   1.000000000
```

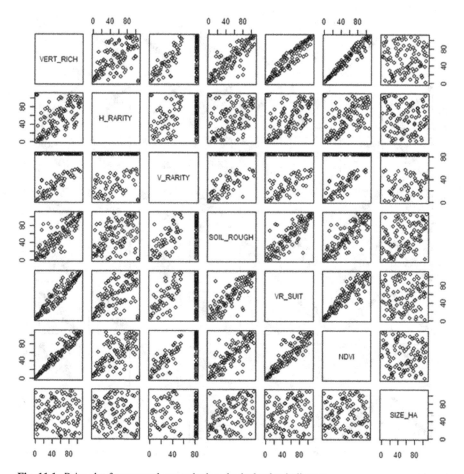

Fig. 11.1 Pairs plot for seven place-ranked ecological value indicators

Ecological value indicator #1 is strongly correlated with indicators #5 and #6, and is also substantially correlated with indicator #4.

Ecological Sensitivity Indicators

There were again nine indicators provided for ecological sensitivity. Eight of these were considered to increase with sensitivity, and one as being contrary. For present purposes, a decision was made here to drop one of the indicators due to a preponderance of zeros. The remaining indicators oriented with sensitivity were then place-ranked, and the counter-indicator was given regular ranks—this latter being the

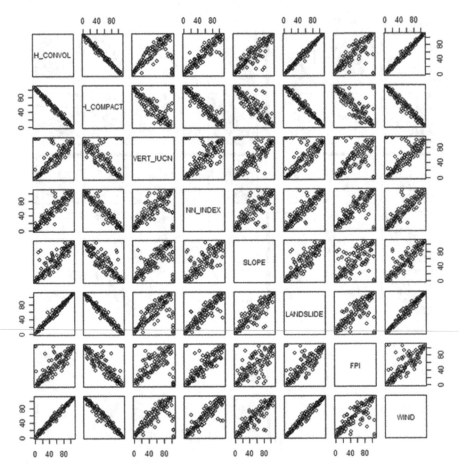

Fig. 11.2 Pairs plot for place-ranked ecological value indicators, the second of which is not carried forward

second indicator. These were then written to a file having EcoSntvR.txt as its name. Pairs plots were then prepared as follows and depicted in Fig. 11.2.

```
@ EcoSntvR <- read.table("EcoSntvR.txt",header=T)
@ pairs(EcoSntvR[,-1])
```

From Fig. 11.2 it can be seen that the reorientation of indicator #2 did not make it consonant with the others, and that it is very strongly correlated with indicator #1 as shown in the correlation matrix for ranks that follows. Due to this inconsistency of indicator #2 along with its informational redundancy to indicator #1, it has been decided here to drop it. Dropping of indicator #2 leaves seven indicators for sensitivity. This is a like number to that for ecological value.

The last indicator is strongly correlated with two of the other remaining indicators.

```
@ cor(EcoSntvR[,-1])
            H_CONVOL  H_COMPACT  VERT_IUCN   NN_INDEX      SLOPE  LANDSLIDE
H_CONVOL   1.0000000 -0.9925715  0.6306710  0.9230615  0.8715420  0.9893109
H_COMPACT -0.9925715  1.0000000 -0.6183860 -0.9460472 -0.8591306 -0.9854311
VERT_IUCN  0.6306710 -0.6183860  1.0000000  0.5880089  0.6869966  0.6271218
NN_INDEX   0.9230615 -0.9460472  0.5880089  1.0000000  0.7778834  0.9062563
SLOPE      0.8715420 -0.8591306  0.6869966  0.7778834  1.0000000  0.8620676
LANDSLIDE  0.9893109 -0.9854311  0.6271218  0.9062563  0.8620676  1.0000000
FPI        0.7705583 -0.7848266  0.4419105  0.7866491  0.6243164  0.7399629
WIND       0.9896253 -0.9768187  0.6430201  0.9014400  0.8839026  0.9819276
                 FPI       WIND
H_CONVOL   0.7705583  0.9896253
H_COMPACT -0.7848266 -0.9768187
VERT_IUCN  0.4419105  0.6430201
NN_INDEX   0.7866491  0.9014400
SLOPE      0.6243164  0.8839026
LANDSLIDE  0.7399629  0.9819276
FPI        1.0000000  0.7524990
WIND       0.7524990  1.0000000
```

For purposes of salient scaling to be conducted, the substantial redundancy in both the ecological value and ecological sensitivity constellations of indicators does not entail impairment to the prioritization process. It should, however, be noted for whatever further work may be done in this context.

Human Pressure Indicators

Six indicators were provided for human pressure, with three being directly indicative and three being counter-indicative. Place-ranking was applied to the three direct indicators, and regular ranking was applied to the three counter-indicators. Thus, better-placed cases have lower rank numbers for all indicators. The resultant rankings were written to a file having HumPresR.txt as its name. Indicators #2 and #3 are very strongly correlated as seen in the following matrix.

```
@ cor(HumPresR[,-1])
           POP_DENS  MEAN_AGE  AGE_RATE DEP_RATIO  NAT_INCR  NET_MIGR
POP_DENS  1.0000000 0.6685768 0.6420508 0.7002489 0.6557695 0.4380636
MEAN_AGE  0.6685768 1.0000000 0.9819274 0.9221818 0.7810924 0.4070985
AGE_RATE  0.6420508 0.9819274 1.0000000 0.8889429 0.7701065 0.3985224
DEP_RATIO 0.7002489 0.9221818 0.8889429 1.0000000 0.7192074 0.3641010
NAT_INCR  0.6557695 0.7810924 0.7701065 0.7192074 1.0000000 0.3412470
NET_MIGR  0.4380636 0.4070985 0.3985224 0.3641010 0.3412470 1.0000000
```

Pairs plots were produced as follows and appear in Fig. 11.3.

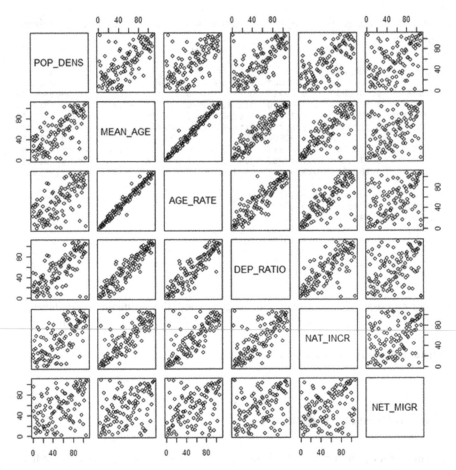

Fig. 11.3 Pairs plot for human pressure indicators (low rank values reflect high pressure)

```
@ HumPresR <- read.table("HumPresR.txt",header=T)
@ pairs(HumPresR[,-1])
```

Salient Scaling

Salient scaling as set forth previously is next conducted for each constellation separately using the salient function given in Chap. 10. The ten most salient cases (communes) are listed for each as returned directly from the function. A data frame of salient scale values arranged in case order is also prepared for use in cross-comparisons among the constellations.

```
@ IDs <- EcoValuR[,1]
@ source("Salient.txt")
@ SalntValu <- Salient(EcoValuR[,-1],IDs)
@ CaseOrdr <- order(SalntValu[,1])
@ SalntValus <- SalntValu[CaseOrdr,]
@ SalntValu[1:10,]
        CaseIDs Salnt
  [1,]      108     1
  [2,]        7     2
  [3,]       19     3
  [4,]      101     4
  [5,]       18     5
  [6,]       11     6
  [7,]       33     7
  [8,]      105     8
  [9,]        9     9
 [10,]        6    10

@ SalntSntv <- Salient(EcoSntvR[,-1],IDs)
@ CaseOrdr <- order(SalntSntv[,1])
@ SalntSntvs <- SalntSntv[CaseOrdr,]
@ SalntSntv[1:10,]
        CaseIDs Salnt
  [1,]       26     1
  [2,]       43     2
  [3,]       94     3
  [4,]       40     4
  [5,]       58     5
  [6,]       18     6
  [7,]       33     7
  [8,]       41     8
  [9,]       17     9
 [10,]       19    10

@ SalntHumn <- Salient(HumPresR[,-1],IDs)
@ CaseOrdr <- order(SalntHumn[,1])
@ SalntHumns <- SalntHumn[CaseOrdr,]
@ SalntHumn[1:10,]
        CaseIDs Salnt
  [1,]        4     1
  [2,]       39     2
  [3,]      104     3
  [4,]      108     4
  [5,]       43     5
  [6,]       17     6
  [7,]       51     7
  [8,]       20     8
  [9,]        8     9
 [10,]       94    10
```

Perusal of the top-ten listings shows that human pressure has one case in common with ecological value and three cases in common with ecological sensitivity. However, there is no case that appears in all three listings. Proceeding with cross-plots of case-ordered salient scores, Fig. 11.4 shows human pressure in relation to ecological value with commune 108 being strongly salient in both respects.

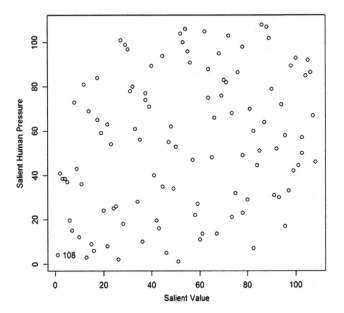

Fig. 11.4 Salient scores of human pressure versus ecological value

```
@ plot(SalntValus[,2],SalntHumns[,2],xlab="Salient Value",
@@ ylab="Salient Human Pressure")
@ identify(SalntValus[,2],SalntHumns[,2])
[1] 108
```

Plotting salient scores of human pressure and ecological sensitivity in Fig. 11.5 highlights the three cases (43, 17 and 94) noted in the listings, along with case 33 and possibly case 6.

```
@ plot(SalntSntvs[,2],SalntHumns[,2],xlab="Salient Sensitive",
@@ ylab="Salient Human Pressure")
@ identify(SalntSntvs[,2],SalntHumns[,2])
```

Salient scores for ecological value and ecological sensitivity are plotted together in Fig. 11.6. This highlights 18, 19, and 33 which appeared in the top ten for both, along with seven which appeared in the top ten only for ecological value and 26 which appeared in the top ten only for ecological sensitivity. Notably, case 33 is also highlighted in the relation of human pressure to ecological sensitivity. Thus, case 33 has prominence in all three regards.

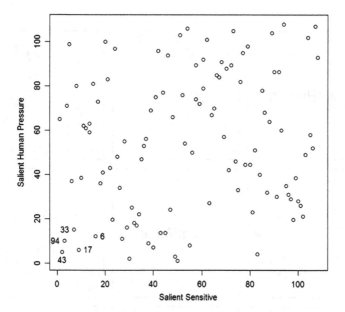

Fig. 11.5 Salient scores of human pressure versus ecological sensitivity

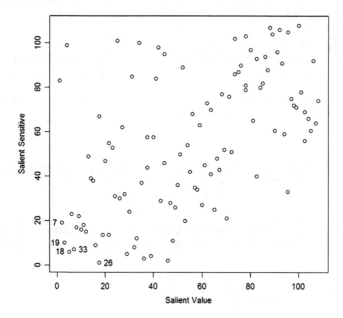

Fig. 11.6 Salient scores of ecological sensitivity versus ecological value

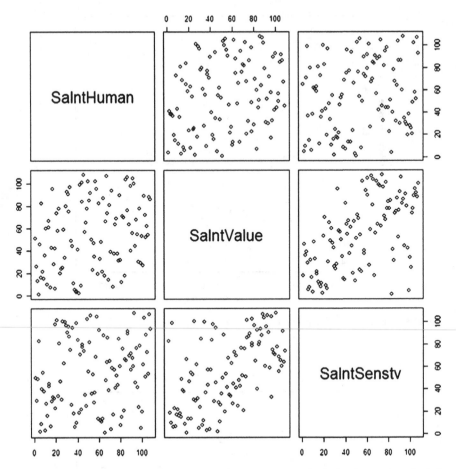

Fig. 11.7 Pairs plot of salient scores for human pressure, ecological value, and ecological sensitivity

```
@ plot(SalntValus[,2],SalntSntvs[,2],xlab="Salient Value",
@@ ylab="Salient Sensitive")
@ identify(SalntValus[,2],SalntSntvs[,2])
```

Pairs plots are frequently helpful in visualizing multiple interrelations. This can be obtained by binding together the three salient scorings and plotting as in Fig. 11.7.

```
@ SalntHuman <- SalntHumns[,2]
@ SalntValue <- SalntValus[,2]
@ SalntSenstv <- SalntSntvs[,2]
@ Salnts <- cbind(SalntHuman,SalntValue,SalntSenstv)
@ pairs(Salnts)
```

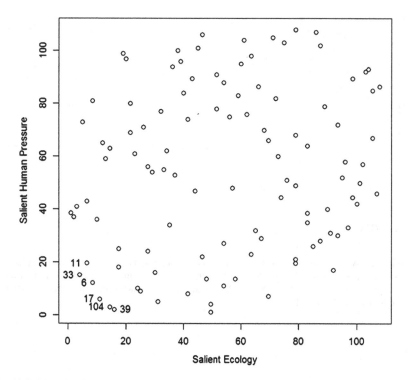

Fig. 11.8 Plot of salient human pressure versus joint salience for ecology

Figure 11.7 reflects association between ecological value and ecological sensitivity, but little for either of these with human pressure—as anticipated earlier.

One further avenue for continuing the investigation is to bind together the ecological value indicators with the ecological sensitivity indicators for joint scoring on a salient scale. Human pressure can then be plotted against the joint salient scores for identifying the interesting elements as in Fig. 11.8. This reinforces a focus on the commune identified as number 33. Commune 17 also appears from the top ten lists for both human pressure and ecological sensitivity. Because of the overall oppositional nature between ecology and human pressure with human pressure tending to pose threats to ecology, it makes less sense to extract joint salient scaling for all three. One should never lose sight of sensibility in pursuing prioritization.

```
@ EcoLogic <- cbind(EcoValuR,EcoSntvR[,-1])
@ SalntEcol <- Salient(EcoLogic[,-1],IDs)
@ CaseOrdr <- order(SalntEcol[,1])
@ SalntEcols <- SalntEcol[CaseOrdr,]
@ plot(SalntEcols[,2],SalntHumns[,2],xlab="Salient Ecology",
@@ ylab="Salient Human Pressure")
@ identify(SalntEcols[,2],SalntHumns[,2])
```

```
@ SalntEcol[1:10,]
       CaseIDs Salnt
 [1,]       19  1.0
 [2,]       18  2.0
 [3,]        7  3.0
 [4,]       33  4.0
 [5,]      105  5.0
 [6,]        9  6.5
 [7,]       11  6.5
 [8,]        6  8.5
 [9,]       25  8.5
[10,]        1 10.0
```

Reference

Rossi F, Pecci A, Amadio V, Rossi O, Soliani L (2008) Coupling indicators of ecological value and
    ecological sensitivity with indicators of demographic pressure in the demarcation of new areas
    to be protected: the case of the Oltrepo Pavese and the Ligurian-Emilian Apennine area (Italy).
    Landsc Urban Plann 86:12–26

Chapter 12
Severity Setting for Human Health

In this chapter, we consider a context of indicators for infant health on the Indonesian island of Java as studied by Ms. Yekti Widyaningsih in cooperation with the authors of this volume. This complements the foregoing material by presenting a setting wherein the indicators are intended to reflect severity of a context of concern instead of favorability. Instead of reversing ratings, we invert interpretations so that previously preferential positions become particularly problematic positions in salient scaling and preference plots. The data pertain to Java Island in 2007 at the district level, omitting Banten Province and Kepulauan District due to incompleteness of information (see Fig. 12.1).

We begin with four indicators as follows: number of infant deaths (infd); thousands of people in poverty (pov); number of infants with low birth weight (lbw); and percentage of births without health personnel present (abhp). These indicators are all seen as increasing concern for infant health. The data file also contained an additional column that is deemed here not to be of present interest.

W.L. Myers and G.P. Patil, *Multivariate Methods of Representing Relations*
in R for Prioritization Purposes, Environmental and Ecological Statistics 6,
DOI 10.1007/978-1-4614-3122-0_12, © Springer Science+Business Media, LLC 2012

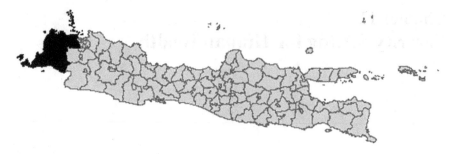

Fig. 12.1 Java Island with excluded areas in *black*

Data Files

The data were extracted from an Excel© spreadsheet into a textual file for access via the read.table() command in **R** as follows:

```
@ JavaData <-read.table("JavHelth.txt",header=T)
@ length(JavaData)
[1] 7
@ JavaData <- JavaData[,-7]
@ names(JavaData)
[1] "District" "CaseIDs" "infd"      "pov"      "lbw"      "abhp"
@ head(JavaData)
  District CaseIDs infd   pov lbw  abhp
1  Pacitan       1   61 125.6 145 20.20
2    Ponor       2  112 157.9 187 14.63
3 Trengglk       3   78 149.1 130 16.19
4   Tulung       4   97 170.5 252  2.95
5   Blitar       5   83 171.2 250  0.51
6   Kediri       6  298 267.4 401 11.56
@ tail(JavaData)
     District CaseIDs infd   pov  lbw  abhp
103   kbanjar     103   69  12.9  105 25.77
104    Jaksel     104  266  35.4  947 14.62
105    Jaktim     105   54 122.6 1962 12.61
106    JakPus     106    6  70.7  129  0.00
107    JakBar     107   22  94.0  610  0.00
108     Jakut     108  108 171.8 1456  8.91
```

The tail() command shows that 108 districts are represented in the data. The first column is an abbreviated district name and the second is a number assigned to the district.

We proceed to convert the data to place-based ranks in which rank 1 indicates the greatest severity and the data frame contains only the ranked indicators.

```
@ JavaRnks <- PlacRank(JavaData[,3:6])
@ head(JavaRnks)
   infd pov  lbw abhp
1 85.5  77 82.0   30
2 53.0  71 71.0   44
3 75.5  72 86.5   41
4 62.0  67 55.0   92
5 72.0  66 56.5   98
6 12.0  40 38.0   59
```

Indicator Screening

The work of Yekti suggests that the last indicator may be of questionable value, so we begin with a pairs() lattice of scatterplots for the indicator ranks (Fig. 12.2).

```
@ pairs(JavaRnks)
```

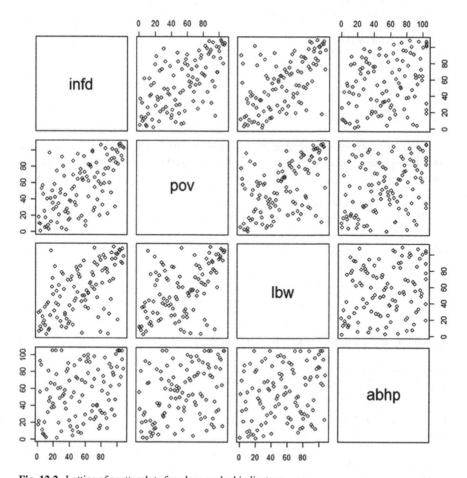

Fig. 12.2 Lattice of scatterplots for place-ranked indicators

Relations are visually evident in Fig. 12.2 among the first three indicators, but not so for the fourth indicator. Therefore, the abhp column is removed before proceeding and rank correlations calculated for the remaining three as follows.

```
@ JavaRnks <- JavaRnks[,-4]
@ cor(JavaRnks)
            infd        pov        lbw
infd 1.0000000 0.6230966 0.6002410
pov  0.6230966 1.0000000 0.5219244
lbw  0.6002410 0.5219244 1.0000000
```

Salient Scaling

We proceed directly to an integrated view of the indicators as reflected in salient scaling, noting that the file of salient scores is arranged in decreasing order of severity.

```
@ CasIDs <- JavaData[,2]
@ JavSalnt <- Salient(JavaRnks,CasIDs)
@ head(JavSalnt)
      CaseIDs Salnt
[1,]      44   1.0
[2,]      83   2.5
[3,]      87   2.5
[4,]      45   4.0
[5,]      90   5.0
[6,]      61   6.0
```

It will be informative to append the salient scores to the file of place-based ranks, but this requires a file of salient scores that is arranged in case order like the file of ranks.

```
@ CaseOrder <- order(JavSalnt[,1])
@ JavSalnts <- JavSalnt[CaseOrder,]
@ head(JavSalnts)
      CaseIDs Salnt
[1,]       1    79
[2,]       2    58
[3,]       3    76
[4,]       4    51
[5,]       5    57
[6,]       6    22
```

Appending is then done in the following manner:

```
@ Salnts <- JavSalnts[,2]
@ JavaRnks <- cbind(JavaRnks,Salnts)
@ head(JavaRnks)
   infd pov  lbw Salnts
1 85.5  77 82.0     79
2 53.0  71 71.0     58
3 75.5  72 86.5     76
4 62.0  67 55.0     51
5 72.0  66 56.5     57
6 12.0  40 38.0     22
```

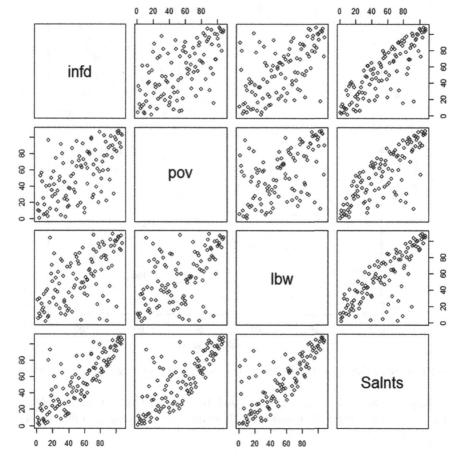

Fig. 12.3 Lattice of scatterplots for salient scores versus individual indicators

The last row and column of a `pairs()` lattice plot (Fig. 12.3) now shows the correspondence or lack thereof between the salient scores and the place-based ranks of the respective indicators.

```
@ pairs(JavaRnks)
```

The plotted points in the lower-right corner of the scattergrams in the last column show districts in which the ranking for an indicator is more severe than the composite salient score might suggest. The scattergram for infant deaths is expanded and tagged with case numbers in Fig. 12.4.

```
@ plot(JavaRnks$Salnts,JavaRnks$infd)
@ identify(JavaRnks$Salnts,JavaRnks$infd)
```

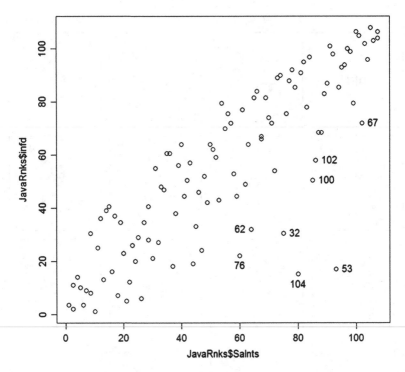

Fig. 12.4 Scatterplot of infant deaths versus salient score, with *line numbers* for selected points

Line numbers 53 (Klaten District) and 104 (Jacsel District) are notable in Fig. 12.4 for the infant death indicator. These lines are extracted from the ranking file as follows:

```
@ JavaRnks[c(53,104),]
     infd pov lbw Salnts
53     17  12 103     93
104    15  96   8     80
```

It can be seen that Klaten District is quite severe with respect to infant death and poverty, but is very well situated with regard to low birth weight which keeps the salient score from reflecting the severity of the other two indicators. Jacsel District is relatively well situated with respect to poverty which keeps the salient score from reflecting the severity of the other two indicators. A low (severe) salient score thus shows an overall context of severity for the district across the indicators.

The corresponding plot of poverty versus salient scores is shown in Fig. 12.5 with tagging of line numbers.

```
@ plot(JavaRnks$Salnts,JavaRnks$pov)
@ identify(JavaRnks$Salnts,JavaRnks$pov)
```

It can be seen that Klaten District also shows here as the most notable outlier, which is consist with the observations from Fig. 12.4. Districts 26, 27, and 29 are Bangk, Sampang, and Sumen, respectively. In these three districts, poverty is more severe than the other two indicators.

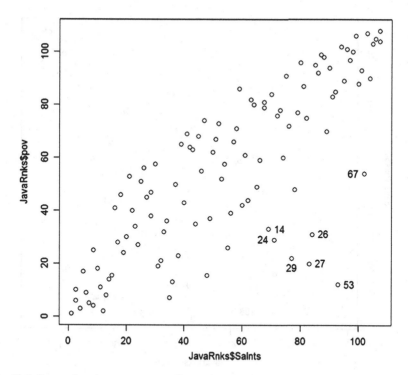

Fig. 12.5 Scatterplot of poverty versus salient score, with *line numbers* for selected points

Likewise, the plot of low birth weight versus salient scores is shown in Fig. 12.6 with tagging of line numbers.

```
@ plot(JavaRnks$Salnts,JavaRnks$lbw)
@ identify(JavaRnks$Salnts,JavaRnks$lbw)
```

There are more places of note for low birth weight than for the other two indicators. Accordingly, these are retrieved as follows:

```
@ Cheklbw <- c(8,37,40,49,97,104,105,107,108)
@ Chekname <- JavaData[Cheklbw,1]
@ Chekdata <- JavaRnks[Cheklbw,]
@ LBWchek <- cbind(Chekname,Chekdata)
@ LBWchek
     Chekname   infd   pov lbw Salnts
8       Lumaj   77.0  61.0  22     61
37     Ksurab   79.5  57.5   4     54
40     Bantul   90.0  60.0  26     74
49      Purwo   84.0  59.0  32     66
97      Kband   44.5  86.0  13     59
104    Jaksel   15.0  96.0   8     80
105    Jaktim   89.0  78.0   2     73
107    JakBar  101.0  83.0  19     91
108     Jakut   56.0  65.0   3     39
```

In all of these cases (places), the low birth weight stands out with regard to severity in comparison to the other two indicators.

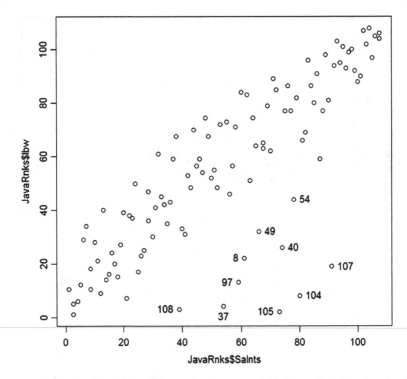

Fig. 12.6 Scatterplot of low birth weight versus salient score, with *line numbers* for selected points

First Quartile of Severity

With 108 districts under consideration, there are 27 districts in each quartile. The first quartile of severity can be taken from the beginning of the JavSalnt file with the corresponding district names and ranks added.

```
> Q1indx <- JavSalnt[1:27,1]
> Q1namID <- JavaData[Q1indx,1:2]
> Q1ranks <- JavaRnks[Q1indx,]
> Q1status <- cbind(Q1namID,Q1ranks)
> Q1status
     District CaseIDs infd   pov   lbw Salnts
44    Cilacap      44  3.5   1.0  10.5    1.0
83      Garut      83 11.0   6.0   1.0    2.5
87    Cirebon      87  2.0  10.0   5.0    2.5
45     Banyum      45 14.0   3.0   6.0    4.0
90     Indram      90 10.0  17.0  12.0    5.0
61       Pati      61  3.5   9.0  29.0    6.0
58       Grob      58  9.0   5.0  34.0    7.0
79      Bogor      79 30.5   4.0  10.5    8.5
84      Tasik      84  8.0  25.0  18.0    8.5
47     Banjar      47  1.0  18.0  28.0   10.0
81    Cianjur      81 25.0  11.0  21.0   11.0
72     Brebes      72 36.0   2.0   9.0   12.0
9      Jember       9 13.0   8.0  40.0   13.0
64      Demak      64 39.0  14.0  14.0   14.0
```

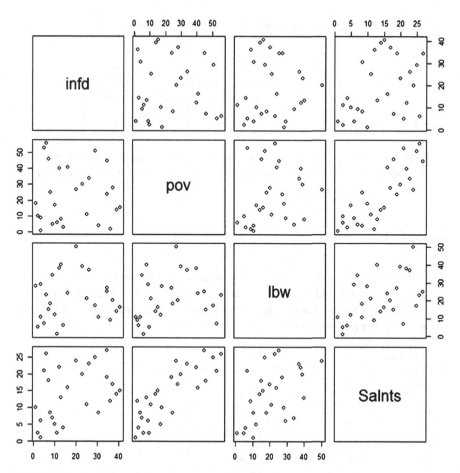

Fig. 12.7 Lattice of scatterplots showing salient scores versus place-based ranks of individual indicators for first quartile of severity

```
7       Malang       7 40.5 15.5 16.0    15.0
17     Jombang      17 16.0 41.0 24.0    16.0
23       Tuban      23 37.0 28.0 20.0    17.0
88       Majal      88  7.0 46.0 15.0    18.0
70       Pemal      70 34.5 24.0 27.0    19.0
93       Karaw      93 23.0 30.0 39.0    20.0
15    Sidoarjo      15  5.0 53.0  7.0    21.0
6       Kediri       6 12.0 40.0 38.0    22.0
13     Proboli      13 26.0 34.0 37.0    23.0
52       Boyol      52 20.0 27.0 50.0    24.0
65       Semar      65 29.0 51.0 17.0    25.0
85      Ciamis      85  6.0 56.0 23.0    26.0
91      Subang      91 34.5 45.0 25.0    27.0
```

A `pairs()` lattice plot for the first quartile of severity is given in Fig. 12.7.

```
@ pairs(Q1status[3:6])
```

The correlation matrix corresponding to Fig. 12.7 is as follows:

```
@ cor(Q1status[3:6])
                 infd           pov          lbw      Salnts
infd      1.000000000  -0.007290827   0.03489347   0.3870166
pov      -0.007290827   1.000000000   0.22255105   0.8334628
lbw       0.034893467   0.222551051   1.00000000   0.5010051
Salnts    0.387016632   0.833462796   0.50100512   1.0000000
```

From Fig. 12.7 and the correlation matrix, it can be seen that the salient score most closely tracks poverty in this subset of severe districts. Low birth weight is next, and infant death is least so.

Precedence

The salient scores provide a sequencing of severity, but offer no further comparative context. Precedence and progression plots offer additional interpretive insights. Toward this end ascribed advantage and subordinate status are obtained according to product-order rating via the ProdOrdr() function.

```
@ PlacBasd <- 1
@ JavaProdOr <- ProdOrdr(CasIDs,JavaRnks[,1:3],PlacBasd)
@ head(JavaProdOr)
        CaseIDs     AA      SS     ORDIT  Salnt
[1,]          1  13.08  57.94  8692.667     79
[2,]          2  19.63  38.32  8037.477     58
[3,]          3  14.02  53.27  8598.620     76
[4,]          4  24.30  35.51  7570.469     51
[5,]          5  20.56  37.38  7944.471     57
[6,]          6  46.73   7.48  5327.140     22
```

A precedence plot can then be constructed as shown in Fig. 12.8.

```
@ TrpzTrpl(JavaProdOr)
@ identify(JavaProdOr[,3],JavaProdOr[,2])
```

A progression plot (Fig. 12.9) can detect any ties in the precedence plot.

```
@ ORDITrank <- rank(JavaProdOr[,4])
@ ORDITstep <- rank(JavaProdOr[,4],ties.method="first")
@ plot(ORDITstep,ORDITrank)
@ identify(ORDITstep,ORDITrank)
```

Examining the precedence plot along with ties, districts with case ids 44, 83, 87, and 45 stand out with regard to severity. Retrieving these and coupling names with ranks, these districts are seen to be Cilacap, Garut, Cirebon, and Banyumas.

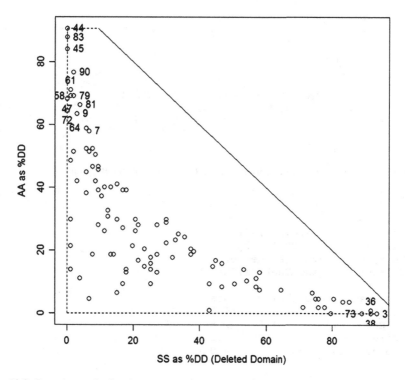

Fig. 12.8 Precedence plot for all districts with selected *line labels*

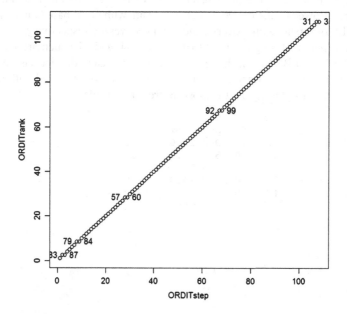

Fig. 12.9 Progression plot showing ties in precedence plot

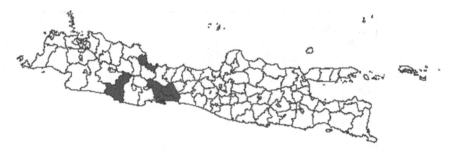

Fig. 12.10 Most notably severe districts Cilacap, Garut, Cirebon, and Banyum

```
@ Chekset <- c(44,83,87,45)
@ Cheknam <- JavaData[Chekset,1]
@ Chekrnk <- JavaRnks[Chekset,]
@ Cheking <- cbind(Cheknam,Chekrnk)
@ Cheking
   Cheknam infd pov  lbw Salnts
44 Cilacap  3.5   1 10.5    1.0
83   Garut 11.0   6  1.0    2.5
87  Cirebon  2.0 10  5.0    2.5
45  Banyum 14.0   3  6.0    4.0
```

There are no place-based ranks with magnitude greater than 14 among this set, so these districts lie in the most severe 13% of rankings on all three indicators. These are followed by district 90, which is Indram, with place-based rankings of 10, 17, and 12 for infant death, poverty, and low birth weight, respectively.

There is next a close grouping of 61, 58, 79, 84, and 47 which are Pati, Grob, Bogor, Tasik, and Banjar. In this group, we find that each district has one place-based ranking of 25 or larger. District 81 (Cianjur) is not far behind with rankings of 25, 11, and 21 rounding out the most severe 10% (decile).

```
   District CaseIDs infd  pov  lbw Salnts
61     Pati      61  3.5  9.0 29.0    6.0
58     Grob      58  9.0  5.0 34.0    7.0
79    Bogor      79 30.5  4.0 10.5    8.5
84    Tasik      84  8.0 25.0 18.0    8.5
47   Banjar      47  1.0 18.0 28.0   10.0
```

At the other extreme of districts without concerns are Trengglk, Kblitar, Kmadiun, Kbatu, and Kmagel.

```
@ Chekset <- c(3,31,36,38,73)
@ Cheknam <- JavaData[Chekset,1]
@ Chekrnk <- JavaRnks[Chekset,]
@ Cheking <- cbind(Cheknam,Chekrnk)
@ Cheking
     Cheknam  infd pov   lbw Salnts
3   Trengglk  75.5  72  86.5   76.0
31   Kblitar 106.5 104 106.0  107.5
36   Kmadiun 102.0 107 102.0  103.0
38     Kbatu 103.0 105 105.0  106.0
73    Kmagel 108.0 103  97.0  105.0
```

The most notably severe districts are mapped in Fig. 12.10.

Part III
Transformation Techniques
and Virtual Variates

Chapter 13
Matrix Methods for Multiple Measures

We return now to the context of Chap. 3 where rotational rescaling was introduced and then exploited in the manner of principal components via the princomp() function facility of **R**. We generalize that work to encompass *linear transformation* of multiple measures to generate a secondary set of what we will call *virtual variates*. We reserve the term virtual variates for situations in which the transformation is reversible so that the original multiple measures can be reproduced from the secondary set through a suitable transformation. In such circumstances, the transformation effectively provides a particular perspective from which to view the data without loss of information. With principal components, the perspective was one of independent (uncorrelated) dimensions (Raykov 2008; Timm 2002; Hair et al. 2010). In the earlier venture, we did not undertake to reverse the principal component transformation, but will do so in the course of current consideration. Virtual variates from principal components are also not the only interesting perspectives of this nature to be explored (Johnson and Wichern 2007; Sengupta 2003; Mukhopadhyay 2009), and linear transformations will entail several additional operators in **R**.

Returning to the very beginning of Chap. 1, we consider a *multivariate data matrix* comprising *p* variates determined on *n* cases in a row/column arrangement with cases as rows and variates as columns. Further, the term *matrix* will apply to any row/column array of values in which there is no missing data. Any single row or column of values constitutes a *vector*, with at least a formal distinction between row vectors and column vectors. For general purposes of presentation, we will consider **X** to be a matrix of data on original variates with $\mathbf{X}^{n \times p}$ indicating that there are *n* rows and *p* columns being the *order* of the matrix so that the multiplication $n \times p$ gives the total number of values, entries, or *elements* in the matrix. The order will often be omitted if it is clear from context. Also $x_{i,j}$ is used to denote the element in row **i** and column **j** without actually specifying a numeric value. Similarly, $\mathbf{X}_I$ denotes the *I*th row of **X** and $\mathbf{X}_J$ denotes the *J*th column.

With this notation, the (inner) product of two vectors **A** and **B** is:

$$a_1 b_1 + a_2 b_2 + \ldots + a_k b_k,$$

W.L. Myers and G.P. Patil, *Multivariate Methods of Representing Relations in R for Prioritization Purposes*, Environmental and Ecological Statistics 6, DOI 10.1007/978-1-4614-3122-0_13, © Springer Science+Business Media, LLC 2012

where both vectors have k elements and **A** is formally a row vector with **B** being a column vector. Less formally, both vectors must have the same number of elements to be *conformable* and the result is the sum of products of corresponding elements. The operator is %*% for simple vector multiplication in **R**.

```
@ A <- c(1,3,5,7)
@ B <- c(2,4,6,8)
@ A %*% B
       [,1]
[1,]   100
@ B %*% A
       [,1]
[1,]   100
```

It can be seen from this simple example that **R** does not make a distinction between row vectors and column vectors for doing simple vector multiplication, and that the result is treated as being a **matrix** having one row and one column.

Referring back to the beginning of Chap. 3, it can be seen that a weighted linear composite of variates for a case has this form:

$$c_1 x_{i1} + c_2 x_{i2} + \ldots + c_p x_{ip},$$

with one vector being a vector of weight coefficients and the other being a vector of variate values for the particular (ith) case. Thus, one (tedious) way of obtaining the weighted composite for all cases would be to extract each case as a vector and do vector multiplications as many times as there are cases.

It should be possible, however, to have the case vectors stacked and do all of the vector products in one operation.

```
@ A1 <- c(1,3,5,7)
@ A2 <- c(2,4,6,8)
@ A <- rbind(A1,A2)
@ A
    [,1] [,2] [,3] [,4]
A1     1    3    5    7
A2     2    4    6    8
@ C <- c(0.1,0.2,0.3,0.4)
@ A %*% C
     [,1]
A1      5
A2      6
@ C %*% A
Error in C %*% A : non-conformable arguments
```

It can be seen by example that **R** is OK with this if the case vectors are stacked in a matrix as rows and the matrix is the first operand with the weight vector as the second, but not if the operands are reversed with the weight vector first and the matrix second. Thus, **R** is making a distinction between row and column layouts when a matrix is involved. This illustrates that such multiplication is not commutative (although it is associative and distributive). Next, consider extending the example by including a second weight vector in the scenario.

```
@ A1 <- c(1,3,5,7)
@ A2 <- c(2,4,6,8)
@ A <- rbind(A1,A2)
@ A
    [,1] [,2] [,3] [,4]
A1    1    3    5    7
A2    2    4    6    8
@ C1 <- c(0.1,0.2,0.3,0.4)
@ C2 <- c(0.4,0.3,0.2,0.1)
@ C <- cbind(C1,C2)
@ C
        C1  C2
[1,]  0.1 0.4
[2,]  0.2 0.3
[3,]  0.3 0.2
[4,]  0.4 0.1
@ A %*% C
     C1 C2
A1    5  3
A2    6  4
```

It can now be seen that **R** extends the vector multiplication scenario to matrices by doing pairs of vector products whereby each row of the first operand is treated as a vector and each column of the second operand is treated as a vector, with a multiplication being done for each pairing of a row vector with a column vector. To make the row vectors compatible (conformable) in number of elements with the column vectors, there must be as many *columns* in the first operand as there are *rows* in the second operand.

Linear Transformation and Hybridization

With $X^{n \times p}$ as our data matrix, consider $T^{p \times m}$ as a *transformation matrix* that must necessarily have **p** rows in order to be conformable, with each of the **m** columns generating a transformed variate that is a weighted composite of the **X** variates whereby the kth element is the weight contribution for the kth variate of **X**. Then, $Y = XT$ is the matrix multiplication equation for the matrix of transformed (**Y**) variates.

Although $Y = XT$ is a conventional formulation for such transformations (Giri 2004; Rencher 2002), it is a prescription for problems in **R** because **T** has the default logical value of **TRUE** and **t** is a default matrix transpose operator that interchanges rows and columns of a matrix. Both of these can be redefined by using them differently, but unforeseen consequences are likely to ensue unless this is done very carefully. Therefore, we avoid using **T** and **t** outside their regular **R** context. Thus, it becomes necessary to choose an alternate formulation for transformations. Accordingly, we refer to linear transformations as ***hybridizations*** of the original variates and **H** is used in the notation instead of **T**.

Thus, **Y** = **XH** is a hybridization of original variates where each hybrid variate has the form:

$$h_1 x_{i1} + h_2 x_{i2} + \ldots + h_p x_{ip},$$

with the **h** coefficients showing how *heavily* a hybrid draws on each original variate.

A simple example of three cases on two variates for **X** with **Y**$_{,1}$ being the sum and **Y**$_{,2}$ being the difference is as follows:

```
@ X <- matrix(c(1,3,2,5,4,6),nrow=3,byrow=T)
@ X
     [,1] [,2]
[1,]    1    3
[2,]    2    5
[3,]    4    6
@ H <- matrix(c(1,1,1,-1),nrow=2,byrow=F)
@ H
     [,1] [,2]
[1,]    1    1
[2,]    1   -1
@ Y <- X %*% H
@ Y
     [,1] [,2]
[1,]    4   -2
[2,]    7   -3
[3,]   10   -2
```

In addition to using **H** for hybridization, this example also uses **T** in its logical role and should serve to warn against using **F** in anything other than its logical role as **FALSE**.

Back Transformation by Inverse

Now, consider the possibility of a back (**B**) transformation that reverses **H** to return to the original X data matrix from **Y**. From **YB** = **XHB** it can be seen that the product **HB** must be such as to leave **X** unchanged if used directly as hybridizing transformer for **X**. There is only one type of matrix, called an *identity* matrix, which has this property. An identity matrix is square (same number of rows as columns) with 1.0

everywhere on the upper-left to lower-right diagonal and 0 elsewhere. An identity matrix with **k** rows and **k** columns is denoted by $\mathbf{I}^{k \times k}$, where **k** is the *order* of the identity matrix. A square matrix having nonzero elements only on the upper-left to lower-right diagonal, such as identity matrix is said to be a *diagonal* matrix. An identity matrix is the matrix analog of the number one for multiplication.

```
@ Q <- matrix(c(1,0,0,1),nrow=2,byrow=T)
@ Q
     [,1] [,2]
[1,]    1    0
[2,]    0    1
@ X %*% Q
     [,1] [,2]
[1,]    1    3
[2,]    2    5
[3,]    4    6
```

Therefore, it is necessary that **HB** = **I** if the hybridizing transformation is reversible. If there is a matrix that multiplies **H** to produce **I**, then it is called the "inverse matrix" of **H**, and is designated by $\mathbf{H}^{-1}$. There is an **R** function solve() that returns the inverse of its input argument if the inverse exists. In order for a matrix to have an inverse, it must be square and *non-singular*. A check on validity of an inverse is to do the multiplication which should give the identity $\mathbf{HH}^{-1} = \mathbf{I}$.

```
@ B <- solve(H)
@ Check <- H %*% B
@ round(Check,digits=8)
     [,1] [,2]
[1,]    1    0
[2,]    0    1
@ Y %*% B
     [,1] [,2]
[1,]    1    3
[2,]    2    5
[3,]    4    6
```

Accordingly, **B** is a valid inverse and back-transform for **H** which makes the **Y** variates virtual variates with respect to **X** according to our definition. A point to note is that a prerequisite for a transform to have a back-transform is that the transform must have as many variates as the original data matrix which was transformed.

Transpose, Symmetric, and Orthogonal

Transposition rearranges a matrix so rows become columns and vice versa. The transpose of a matrix **V** is denoted as **V'** and is accomplished with the t() function provided in **R**.

```
@ V <- matrix(c(1,-1,1,1),nrow=2,byrow=T)
@ V
     [,1] [,2]
[1,]    1   -1
[2,]    1    1
@ t(V)
     [,1] [,2]
[1,]    1    1
[2,]   -1    1
```

A (square) matrix that is not changed by transposing is said to be *symmetric*.

```
@ H
     [,1] [,2]
[1,]    1    1
[2,]    1   -1
@ t(H)
     [,1] [,2]
[1,]    1    1
[2,]    1   -1
```

A matrix for which the inverse is the transpose is said to be *orthogonal*. We note that the transpose of a product is the product of transposes. Similarly, the inverse of a product is the product of inverses.

Vector Magnitude, Length, or Norm and Euclidean Distance

It was noted at the beginning of Chap. 3 that a transform vector consists of direction cosines for axial rotation if the sum of its squared elements is 1. The sum of squared elements is obtained as the product of a vector with itself.

```
@ W <- c(0.1,0.2,0.3,0.4)
@ W %*% W
     [,1]
[1,]  0.3
```

If the vector is viewed as a set of coordinates on multiple axes, this is the squared distance from the origin to the point—or the squared length of the line connecting the origin with the point. The magnitude, length, or norm of a vector is the square root of this product. If a vector has length 1.0, then its squared length will be the same. If a vector has length 1.0, then it is said to be *normalized*. This is not to be confused in any respect with the normal or Gaussian distribution. If the length of a vector is *L*, then a normalized version of the vector is obtained by multiplying every element by the reciprocal of the length.

```
@ W
[1] 0.1 0.2 0.3 0.4
@ L <- sqrt(W %*% W)
@ W <- W * (1/L)
@ W %*% W
      [,1]
[1,]    1
@ W
[1] 0.1825742 0.3651484 0.5477226 0.7302967
```

For a hybridization matrix **H**, the squared lengths of the vectors appear on the diagonal of the product matrix **H′H** as follows.

```
@ t(H) %*% H
     [,1] [,2]
[1,]    2    0
[2,]    0    2
```

The diagonal of the matrix can be extracted into a vector using the diag() command. We also note in passing that the sum of diagonal elements in a square matrix is called the *trace* of the matrix.

```
@ L <- diag( t(H) %*% H)
@ L
[1] 2 2
@ L <- sqrt(L)
@ L
[1] 1.414214 1.414214
```

The vector can then be used to create a diagonal matrix **G** as follows.

```
@ G <- diag(L)
@ G
          [,1]       [,2]
[1,] 1.414214 0.000000
[2,] 0.000000 1.414214
```

The inverse of a diagonal matrix is a diagonal matrix of reciprocals (of the elements in the diagonal matrix).

```
@ G <- solve(G)
# G now has reciprocals of previous elements.
@ G
          [,1]       [,2]
[1,] 0.7071068 0.0000000
[2,] 0.0000000 0.7071068
```

Multiplying by a diagonal matrix as second operand will multiply every element of a column in the first operand by the respective diagonal element. This can be used to obtain a normalized version of the transformation vector consisting of direction cosines.

```
@ H %*% G
              [,1]          [,2]
[1,] 0.7071068  0.7071068
[2,] 0.7071068 -0.7071068
```

As stated above, the length of a vector is a special case of the *Euclidean distance* between two points in multidimensional space. The special case is that one of the two points is the origin, for which the coordinates are a vector of zeros. The general procedure for calculating Euclidean distance is to subtract the two vectors of coordinates and then calculate the length of the difference vector. The Euclidean distance computation is illustrated as follows.

```
@ A1
[1] 1 3 5 7
@ A2
[1] 2 4 6 8
@ Adif <- A1 - A2
@ Adif
[1] -1 -1 -1 -1
@ Adist <- sqrt(Adif %*% Adif)
@ Adist
       [,1]
[1,]    2
```

Statistics of Transformation

The vector of means for transformed variates is the transform of the mean vector of original variates. Note recasting matrices as data frames to use the mean() function.

```
@ Xmean <- mean(as.data.frame(X))
@ Xmean
        V1          V2
2.333333 4.666667
@ Ymean <- mean(as.data.frame(Y))
@ Ymean
         V1          V2
 7.000000 -2.333333
@ Xmean %*% H
       [,1]        [,2]
[1,]     7 -2.333333
```

If **C** is the matrix of covariances for original variates, the covariance matrix for transformed variates is **H′CH**.

```
@ Xcov <- cov(as.data.frame(X))
@ Xcov
          V1        V2
V1 2.333333 2.166667
V2 2.166667 2.333333
@ Ycov <- cov(as.data.frame(Y))
@ Ycov
    V1        V2
V1  9 0.0000000
V2  0 0.3333333
@ t(H) %*% Xcov %*% H
     [,1]       [,2]
[1,]    9 0.0000000
[2,]    0 0.3333333
```

If a covariance is zero, then the correlation must also be zero; and the reverse is also true whereby zero correlation also implies zero covariance. Since Ycov is diagonal, these particular Y-variates are therefore uncorrelated (being independent in the sense of nonredundant).

Invariant Vectors, Eigenvalues, Modal Matrix, and Spectral Matrix

The relationship for transformed covariance as **H′CH** as given above raises interest in *invariant vectors* and *eigenvalues*. As a point of departure for this exploration, which will lead us back to principal components, we note that a covariance matrix is square and symmetric.

A square matrix **G** may have an associated column-wise matrix of *invariant vectors* **V** such that **GV = VE** with **E** being a diagonal matrix of scaling factors that change the length but not the direction of the vectors. This lack of directional change is why the vectors are called *invariant*. Invariant vectors are also called *characteristic vectors*, *eigenvectors*, or *latent vectors* for the matrix **G**. That is, multiplying the matrix **G** by an invariant vector as second operand gives the same vector with its length changed by the factor in the corresponding position of the diagonal of **E**. We recall that changing the length of a vector consists of multiplying each of its elements by the same (constant) factor. These factors on the diagonal of **E** are called *eigenvalues*. In other words, these are characteristic vector *directions* that do not undergo directional change as multipliers of the matrix. A matrix of the column-wise eigenvectors is called a *modal matrix* of **G**, and a diagonal matrix of eigenvalues is called a *spectral matrix* of **G**. It is a further property that the modal matrix of normalized eigenvectors for a (real) symmetric **G** matrix is orthogonal, so its transpose is its inverse.

The current interest in modal and spectral matrices stems from the property that $\mathbf{V^{-1}GV = E}$ where we recall that the $\mathbf{E}$ matrix of eigenvalues is diagonal. Further, if $\mathbf{G}$ is symmetric, then $\mathbf{V'GV = E}$. We now notice that a covariance matrix $\mathbf{C}$ is symmetric and will yield eigenvalues and normalized eigenvectors. If we use the eigenvectors as a hybridizing transformation for the parent data matrix, we will have $\mathbf{H'CH = E}$. Thus, variances of the transformed (virtual) variates will be the eigenvalues and these transformed variates will be uncorrelated since all of the transformed covariances are zero. $\mathbf{R}$ makes available the eigen() command with which to obtain the modal and spectral matrices needed.

Decorrelation of Standardized Variates

We now undertake by direct matrix methods to decorrelate the standardized BAMBI data which was accomplished by the princomp() command in Chap. 3. We need the covariance matrix of the standardized data, which is also the correlation matrix due to the unit variances produced by standardization. We then apply the eigen() function to obtain eigenvalues and eigenvectors. Multiletter names are used so that the letter T can be incorporated without conflicts in $\mathbf{R}$

```
@ BAMBIS <- read.table("BAMBIs.txt",header=T)
@ head(BAMBIS)
       BirdSp    MamlSp     ElevSD      PctFor    Pct1FPch    Pct1OPch
1 -4.5219358 -2.679155 -1.6642353 -1.5293840 -0.9866461   2.2794565
2 -4.3199041 -1.959026 -1.0954558  0.6354669  0.7226492  -0.5366323
3 -0.4139576 -1.959026 -1.2308795 -0.8697464 -0.5610808   0.4381677
4 -1.7608357 -2.679155 -1.5017269 -1.9765210 -1.5177234   2.0677576
5 -2.4342748 -1.959026 -0.5808457  1.3305213  1.2853802  -0.9009515
6 -0.2792698 -1.478939 -1.0142016  0.1883300  0.3744595  -0.2953939

@ BSC <- cov(BAMBIS)
@ BSC
             BirdSp     MamlSp     ElevSD      PctFor   Pct1FPch   Pct1OPch
BirdSp    1.0000000  0.5788003  0.3555759  0.2112191  0.1880800 -0.2403293
MamlSp    0.5788003  1.0000000  0.5918184  0.4829511  0.4463258 -0.4517020
ElevSD    0.3555759  0.5918184  1.0000000  0.4532556  0.4233015 -0.4025587
PctFor    0.2112191  0.4829511  0.4532556  1.0000000  0.9708868 -0.8918867
Pct1FPch  0.1880800  0.4463258  0.4233015  0.9708868  1.0000000 -0.8707050
Pct1OPch -0.2403293 -0.4517020 -0.4025587 -0.8918867 -0.8707050  1.0000000

@ BSE <- eigen(BSC)
@ summary(BSE)
          Length Class  Mode
values    6      -none- numeric
vectors   36     -none- numeric
@ attributes(BSE)
$names
[1] "values"  "vectors"
```

The eigenvalues are returned in a $values *vector* and the eigenvectors are returned in a $vectors *matrix*. We transfer these into separate objects for convenience of further work.

```
@ BST <- BSE$vectors
@ BSV <- BSE$values
@ BSV
[1] 3.62316546 1.28251288 0.59990466 0.32198500 0.14549351 0.02693849
@ BST
           [,1]         [,2]         [,3]        [,4]        [,5]         [,6]
[1,] -0.2469913  0.6310407 -0.58550302  0.43764041 -0.08000591  0.006252864
[2,] -0.3824240  0.4507332  0.04123500 -0.80447181  0.03129827 -0.027141967
[3,] -0.3503598  0.3252900  0.78545809  0.39101895  0.03685539 -0.015357738
[4,] -0.4828391 -0.3087169 -0.06525640  0.01530091 -0.32454220  0.749493213
[5,] -0.4717032 -0.3364034 -0.07917502  0.03531989 -0.47578279 -0.656081846
[6,]  0.4629878  0.2904139  0.16737502 -0.08317777 -0.81213562  0.082491760
@ diag(t(BST) %*% BST)
[1] 1 1 1 1 1 1
```

The eigenvalues are the same as those from princomp() in Chap. 3, and the eigen-vectors are the same as principal component loadings except for the reversal of signs on the vector for the third transformed variate. As noted earlier, any constant multiple of an eigenvector is also an eigenvector, so signs can be reversed as desired using −1 as a constant multiplier. The eigenvectors are normalized since they have length = 1.

In the earlier work on principal components, it was decided to the reverse the signs on principal component axes 1, 3, and 5. Here, it will be more convenient to do sign reversals on the transformation vectors before generating the actual trans-formed variates. This is easily done by multiplying the transformation matrix by a suitable diagonal matrix having −1 in positions to be reversed and 1 in positions to remain unchanged.

```
@ #First make the diagonal matrix for changing signs.
@ ReSign <- diag(c(-1,1,1,1,-1,1))
@ #Visually check the diagonal matrix.
@ ReSign
     [,1] [,2] [,3] [,4] [,5] [,6]
[1,]   -1    0    0    0    0    0
[2,]    0    1    0    0    0    0
[3,]    0    0    1    0    0    0
[4,]    0    0    0    1    0    0
[5,]    0    0    0    0   -1    0
[6,]    0    0    0    0    0    1
@ BST <- BST %*% ReSign
@ BST
           [,1]         [,2]         [,3]        [,4]        [,5]         [,6]
[1,]  0.2469913  0.6310407 -0.58550302  0.43764041  0.08000591  0.006252864
[2,]  0.3824240  0.4507332  0.04123500 -0.80447181 -0.03129827 -0.027141967
[3,]  0.3503598  0.3252900  0.78545809  0.39101895 -0.03685539 -0.015357738
[4,]  0.4828391 -0.3087169 -0.06525640  0.01530091  0.32454220  0.749493213
[5,]  0.4717032 -0.3364034 -0.07917502  0.03531989  0.47578279 -0.656081846
[6,] -0.4629878  0.2904139  0.16737502 -0.08317777  0.81213562  0.082491760
```

The transformed variates corresponding to principal component scores can now be generated by multiplying the standardized data matrix by the transformation matrix. Note the need for recasting the data frame of standardized variates as a matrix. Since the computational operations are not being done in exactly the same way (Afifi et al. 2004), some slight differences due to rounding may be expected. Both inverses and eigenvector operations are quite sensitive to numerical rounding/truncation errors. Note carefully that it is standardized data that is being transformed, rather than the original data. Parallel operations for original data will be conducted subsequently.

```
@ BSY <- as.matrix(BAMBIS) %*% BST
@ head(BSY)
          [,1]        [,2]        [,3]        [,4]         [,5]          [,6]
[1,] -4.9837441 -3.1364249  1.7893889 -0.7222740  0.66885632 -0.2409046325
[2,] -1.3038023 -4.5605005  1.3995990 -0.6630448 -0.12968864  0.0008771102
[3,] -2.1701505 -0.9601097 -0.6306928  0.8439480 -0.11981083 -0.1781220052
[4,] -4.6132321 -1.0859814  0.3361935  0.5416484  0.31405080 -0.2302949040
[5,]  0.1119472 -3.7128771  0.5488730  0.4242189  0.19964230  0.1264521048
[6,] -0.5855639 -1.4426438 -0.7854627  0.7116508  0.06070625 -0.0749206244
```

The desired uncorrelated condition can also be checked, again using appropriate recasting of operands.

```
@ round(cov(as.data.frame(BSY)),digits=8)
          V1        V2          V3        V4         V5          V6
V1  3.623165  0.000000  0.0000000  0.000000  0.0000000  0.00000000
V2  0.000000  1.282513  0.0000000  0.000000  0.0000000  0.00000000
V3  0.000000  0.000000  0.5999047  0.000000  0.0000000  0.00000000
V4  0.000000  0.000000  0.0000000  0.321985  0.0000000  0.00000000
V5  0.000000  0.000000  0.0000000  0.000000  0.1454935  0.00000000
V6  0.000000  0.000000  0.0000000  0.000000  0.0000000  0.02693849
```

The variances of the transformed data are equal to the eigenvalues as expected. Since the normalized modal matrix used as a transform is orthogonal, the back transform is its transpose. This is exemplified by doing a back transform on the fifth case, which matches the fifth line of the head() listing of BAMBIS shown earlier in this section.

```
@ Case5Y <- BSY[5,]
@ Case5Y
[1]   0.1119472 -3.7128771  0.5488730  0.4242189  0.1996423  0.1264521
@ Case5Y %*% t(BST)
          [,1]        [,2]        [,3]      [,4]      [,5]        [,6]
[1,] -2.434275 -1.959026 -0.5808457 1.330521 1.285380 -0.9009515
```

It may also be of interest at this juncture to demonstrate that the principal component transformation preserves Euclidean distance between cases as stated in Chap. 3. We do so by calculating the squared distance between cases 4 and 5 for both original and transformed variates.

```
@ Case45X <- as.matrix(BAMBIS[4:5,])
@ Diff45X <- Case45X[1,] - Case45X[2,]
@ Diff45X %*% Diff45X
         [,1]
[1,] 29.42728
@ Case45Y <- as.matrix(BSY[4:5,])
@ Diff45Y <- Case45Y[1,] - Case45Y[2,]
@ Diff45Y %*% Diff45Y
         [,1]
[1,] 29.42728
```

The lines on a biplot serve the purpose of showing the alignment and influence of the original **X** variates on the transformed **Y** variates. This information arises

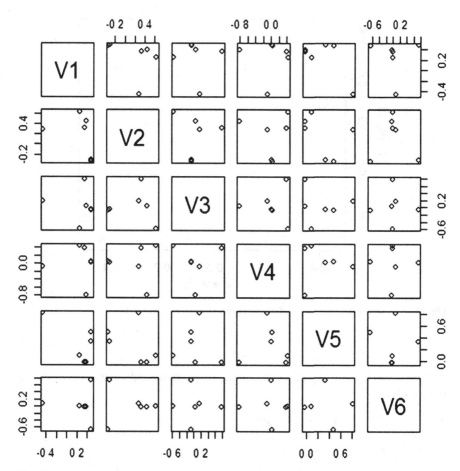

Fig. 13.1 Pairs() plot of transformed **X**-basis vectors in **Y**-space for decorrelating standardized biodiversity data. Each plotted point represents a "pure" **X**-variate as positioned in **Y**-variate space

from transforming a set of basis vectors for **X** as if they were data cases. However, the set of basis vectors takes the form of an identity matrix, and transforming an identity matrix simply gives the transformation matrix. Therefore, the *rows* of the transformation matrix constitute the desired pseudo-cases for **Y**. An alternative to generating lines on plots for pairs of **Y**-axes is to use the pairs() plotting facility for examining this aspect of the information across several of the **Y**-axes as shown in Fig. 13.1 resulting from the command:

```
@ pairs(as.data.frame(BST))
```

Figure 13.1 reflects the correlation structure among the **X**-variates, and thus gives a kind of visual representation of the correlation matrix as a means for interpreting the transformation (loading) matrix.

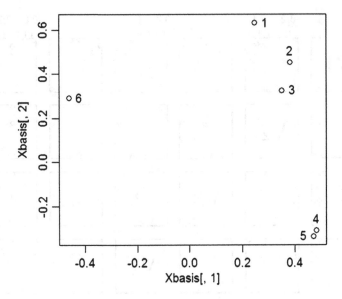

Fig. 13.2 Expansion and labeling of box in *column* one and *row* two of Fig. 13.1

Expansion and labeling of the box in the first column and second row is shown in Fig. 13.2.

```
@ Xbasis <- as.data.frame(BST)
@ plot(Xbasis[,1],Xbasis[,2])
@ identify(Xbasis[,1],Xbasis[,2])
```

The numbers on the points in Fig. 13.2 show the "basis case" that is plotted, and thus the particular basis vector that has been transformed. It shows that BirdSp, MamlSp, and ElevSD are substantially related in this aspect of the first two (major) transformed variates reflecting 82% of the total variance. PctFor and Pct1FPch are very closely related, but rather distant from the first three on transformed axis 2. Pct1OPch opposes all of the others, most particularly on transformed axis 1. Examining the numeric values of the loadings for the first two transformed variates will confirm these interpretations.

We note that multiplying the transformation matrix by a diagonal matrix as second operand will change the variances of the transformed variables, but will not introduce correlations. This is exemplified by using a diagonal matrix to rescale the transformation matrix so that the lengths of the transform vectors are equal to the inverse square roots of the respective eigenvalues.

```
@ Q <- sqrt(BSV)
@ Q <- diag(Q)
@ Q <- solve(Q)
@ Q
            [,1]       [,2]       [,3]       [,4]       [,5]      [,6]
[1,]  0.5253587 0.0000000 0.000000 0.000000 0.000000 0.00000
[2,]  0.0000000 0.8830171 0.000000 0.000000 0.000000 0.00000
[3,]  0.0000000 0.0000000 1.291097 0.000000 0.000000 0.00000
[4,]  0.0000000 0.0000000 0.000000 1.762309 0.000000 0.00000
[5,]  0.0000000 0.0000000 0.000000 0.000000 2.621671 0.00000
[6,]  0.0000000 0.0000000 0.000000 0.000000 0.000000 6.09275
@ BTQ <- BST %*% Q
@ BQY <- as.matrix(BAMBIS) %*% BTQ
@ round(cov(as.data.frame(BQY)),digits=8)
   V1 V2 V3 V4 V5 V6
V1  1  0  0  0  0  0
V2  0  1  0  0  0  0
V3  0  0  1  0  0  0
V4  0  0  0  1  0  0
V5  0  0  0  0  1  0
V6  0  0  0  0  0  1
```

The effect of this rescaling is to produce standardized versions of the transformed variates, which do not reflect the differences in contribution to total variance among the (principal component) variates.

Decorrelation of Original Variates

We now proceed in parallel manner to decorrelate the original BAMBI variates instead of the standardized variates. This is again a version of the principal components idea, but it must take the *covariance* matrix of original variates rather than the correlation matrix as its point of beginning. Consequently, it will be compositing (hybridizing) variates that are not dimensionless and do not have the same units of measure. Therefore, interpretation must be very circumspect unless the original variates have some commonalities among the units in which they are measured— which is not true for the current data.

```
@ BAMBI <- read.table("BAMBI.txt",header=T)
@ head(BAMBI)
  HexNo BirdSp MamlSp ElevSD PctFor Pct1FPch Pct1OPch
1  1714     55     34     11   35.4     35.4     64.6
2  1827     58     37     32   84.3     84.0      7.4
3  1828    116     37     27   50.3     47.5     27.2
4  1829     96     34     17   25.3     20.3     60.3
5  1941     86     37     51  100.0    100.0      0.0
6  1942    118     39     35   74.2     74.1     12.3
@ BAMBI6 <- BAMBI[,-1]
@ head(BAMBI6)
  BirdSp MamlSp ElevSD PctFor Pct1FPch Pct1OPch
1     55     34     11   35.4     35.4     64.6
2     58     37     32   84.3     84.0      7.4
3    116     37     27   50.3     47.5     27.2
4     96     34     17   25.3     20.3     60.3
5     86     37     51  100.0    100.0      0.0
6    118     39     35   74.2     74.1     12.3
@ B6C <- cov(BAMBI6)
@ B6C
               BirdSp     MamlSp      ElevSD      PctFor    Pct1FPch    Pct1OPch
BirdSp      220.49736   35.80478   194.94376    70.84607    79.40788   -72.48667
MamlSp       35.80478   17.35486    91.02787    45.44589    52.86664   -38.22190
ElevSD      194.94376   91.02787  1363.17202   378.00657   444.36957  -301.89381
PctFor       70.84607   45.44589   378.00657   510.22497   623.54617  -409.20433
Pct1FPch     79.40788   52.86664   444.36957   623.54617   808.42241  -502.85167
Pct1OPch    -72.48667  -38.22190  -301.89381  -409.20433  -502.85167   412.57162
@ B6E <- eigen(B6C)
@ summary(B6C)
     BirdSp           MamlSp           ElevSD            PctFor
 Min.   :-72.49   Min.   :-38.22   Min.   :-301.9   Min.   :-409.2
 1st Qu.: 44.57   1st Qu.: 21.97   1st Qu.: 117.0   1st Qu.:  51.8
 Median : 75.13   Median : 40.63   Median : 286.5   Median : 224.4
 Mean   : 88.17   Mean   : 34.05   Mean   : 361.6   Mean   : 203.1
 3rd Qu.:166.06   3rd Qu.: 51.01   3rd Qu.: 427.8   3rd Qu.: 477.2
 Max.   :220.50   Max.   : 91.03   Max.   :1363.2   Max.   : 623.5
    Pct1FPch         Pct1OPch
 Min.   :-502.9   Min.   :-502.85
 1st Qu.: 59.5    1st Qu.:-382.38
 Median : 261.9   Median :-187.19
 Mean   : 251.0   Mean   :-152.01
 3rd Qu.: 578.8   3rd Qu.: -46.79
 Max.   : 808.4   Max.   : 412.57
@ summary(B6E)
         Length Class  Mode
values   6      -none- numeric
vectors  36     -none- numeric
@ B6T <- B6E$vectors
@ B6V <- B6E$values
@ B6V
[1] 2205.801690  840.065521  192.051479   70.194872   16.597700    7.531974
@ B6T
            [,1]        [,2]        [,3]        [,4]        [,5]        [,6]
[1,] -0.11219405 -0.10825381  0.97257848 -0.12600731 -0.02275718 -0.115710722
[2,] -0.05586504 -0.02683217  0.10878243 -0.01447096  0.13541999  0.982739809
[3,] -0.62957347 -0.75900848 -0.15926711  0.02000469 -0.02282496 -0.035442836
[4,] -0.42672854  0.33714474 -0.02849418 -0.16050579  0.81344752 -0.126353834
[5,] -0.52759352  0.45504664 -0.07462183 -0.45283828 -0.54808801  0.059550312
[6,]  0.35703875 -0.30121962 -0.10252380 -0.86757590  0.13610740 -0.008109904
@ diag(t(B6T) %*% B6T)
[1] 1 1 1 1 1 1
```

The eigenvectors are again normalized. The percentages of total variance are:

```
@ B6totl <- sum(B6V)
@ B6pct <- B6V * (100/B6totl)
@ B6pct
[1] 66.1956986 25.2102101  5.7634292  2.1065350  0.4980939  0.2260331
```

Whereas for the standardized scenario they were:

```
@ BStotl <- sum(BSV)
@ BSpct <- BSV * (100/BStotl)
@ BSpct
[1] 60.3860909 21.3752147  9.9984109  5.3664166  2.4248919  0.4489749
```

Since the signs of the transformation coefficients are predominantly negative on all axes, it is appropriate to reverse the directions of all eigenvectors.

```
@ ReSgn <- diag(c(-1,-1,-1,-1,-1,-1))
@ B6T <- B6T %*% ReSgn
@ B6T
            [,1]        [,2]        [,3]        [,4]        [,5]        [,6]
[1,]  0.11219405  0.10825381 -0.97257848  0.12600731  0.02275718  0.115710722
[2,]  0.05586504  0.02683217 -0.10878243  0.01447096 -0.13541999 -0.982739809
[3,]  0.62957347  0.75900848  0.15926711 -0.02000469  0.02282496  0.035442836
[4,]  0.42672854 -0.33714474  0.02849418  0.16050579 -0.81344752  0.126353834
[5,]  0.52759352 -0.45504664  0.07462183  0.45283828  0.54808801 -0.059550312
[6,] -0.35703875  0.30121962  0.10252380  0.86757590 -0.13610740  0.008109904
```

The transformed variates can now be generated by multiplying the *original* data matrix by the transformation matrix with appropriate recasting of operands.

```
@ B6Y <- as.matrix(BAMBI6) %*% B6T
@ head(B6Y)
          [,1]       [,2]        [,3]      [,4]       [,5]       [,6]
[1,]  25.71369   6.630559  -45.16514 84.96015 -21.28782 -23.77045
[2,] 106.36960 -32.856411  -45.90899 65.19282 -26.50165 -22.80657
[3,]  68.89368   3.663539 -104.77740 67.79347 -20.33878 -18.23443
[4,]  23.34973  24.604138  -85.94069 77.81688 -19.69288 -19.22549
[5,] 139.25615 -30.207087  -69.23248 71.68622 -28.42530 -17.92231
[6,] 103.81907 -14.644393 -104.52764 70.86910 -23.21576 -18.36996
```

Since the data were not standardized, the means of the transformed variates are not zero as was the situation with the standardized scenario.

```
@ mean(as.data.frame(B6Y))
        V1         V2         V3         V4         V5         V6
 118.62842   22.47768 -103.56780   70.43304  -26.29270  -22.47256
```

If negative means for transformed data are seen as undesirable, then we would return to the axis reversal step above and change the negatives to positives for 3, 5, and 6 in the diagonal matrix. Alternatively, we could subtract the original mean vector from the original data matrix in order to center the data and then proceed to transform the centered data. The desired uncorrelated condition can again be checked using appropriate recasting of operands.

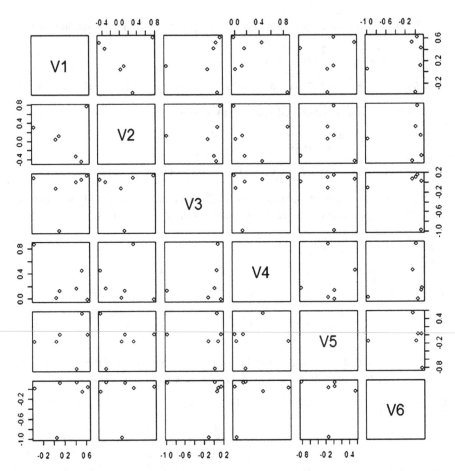

Fig. 13.3 Pairs() plot of transformed **X**-basis vectors in **Y**-space for decorrelating original biodiversity data. Each plotted point represents a "pure" **X**-variate as positioned in **Y**-variate space

```
@ round(cov(as.data.frame(B6Y)),digits=8)
            V1        V2        V3        V4        V5        V6
V1  2205.802    0.0000    0.0000   0.00000    0.0000  0.000000
V2     0.000  840.0655    0.0000   0.00000    0.0000  0.000000
V3     0.000    0.0000  192.0515   0.00000    0.0000  0.000000
V4     0.000    0.0000    0.0000  70.19487    0.0000  0.000000
V5     0.000    0.0000    0.0000   0.00000   16.5977  0.000000
V6     0.000    0.0000    0.0000   0.00000    0.0000  7.531974
```

The variances of the transformed data are again equal to the eigenvalues as expected. Since the normalized modal matrix used as a transform is orthogonal, the back transform is its transpose—which will not be performed for the present purpose. For comparison with the standardized scenario, we explore the biplot relations by a pairs() plot in Fig. 13.3 and then expand and label the box in first column and second row as Fig. 13.4.

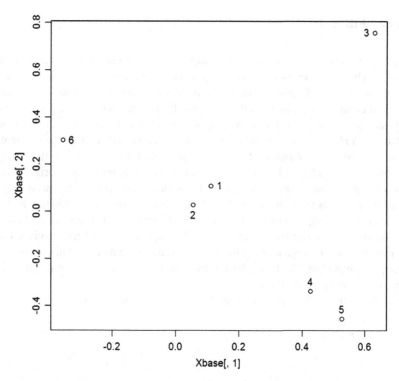

Fig. 13.4 Expansion and labeling of box in *column* one and *row* two of Fig. 13.3

```
@ pairs(as.data.frame(B6T))
@ Xbase <- as.data.frame(B6T)
@ plot(Xbase[,1],Xbase[,2])
@ identify(Xbase[,1],Xbase[,2])
```

Variates 4–6 are similarly situated in Figs. 13.2 and 13.4. However, variate 3 is now strongly segregated from variates 1 and 2; which was not so with respect to standardized variates in Fig. 13.2. Thus, the structural picture for original variates is more in tune with what might be intuitively anticipated; whereby species richness variates stand apart from forest variates, with both being apart from the topographic variate. Further, the deforestation variate is diametrically opposite from the forest cover variates relative to species richness. This type of structural plot is again more intuitively appealing than attempting to interpret the values of transformation coefficients directly, and is simpler that trying to unravel a biplot.

Linear Filter

In doing clustering for contingents in Chap. 4, principal component number 6 was omitted as being an inconsequential component of variation. It is possible to observe directly the extent of perturbation in the data matrix due to omitting one or more principal components, although this is generally not incorporated in presentations on principal components. This can be approached through the back-transform procedure $\mathbf{X} = \mathbf{YH'}$ (expressed in the notation of hybridization) wherein the element in the ith row and jth column of $\mathbf{H'}$ specifies the "contribution" of the ith principal component to the jth original variate. To regenerate the approximated original variates without the contribution of a particular principal component, we need only to set all of the elements in the ith row of $\mathbf{H'}$ to zero—or omit both this row and the corresponding principal component from the back transform. This effectively "filters" the contribution of the particular principal component out of the original data. We illustrate this by regenerating the fifth standardized data case without the sixth principal component. We then plot the filtered data case against the original data case to show the perturbations.

We first remove the sixth row from the back-transform matrix.

```
@ BSF <- t(BST)
@ BSF <- BSF[-6,]
@ BSF
             [,1]          [,2]          [,3]          [,4]          [,5]          [,6]
[1,]   0.24699128    0.38242403    0.35035978    0.48283913    0.47170320   -0.46298775
[2,]   0.63104069    0.45073315    0.32529005   -0.30871693   -0.33640342    0.29041393
[3,]  -0.58550302    0.04123500    0.78545809   -0.06525640   -0.07917502    0.16737502
[4,]   0.43764041   -0.80447181    0.39101895    0.01530091    0.03531989   -0.08317777
[5,]   0.08000591   -0.03129827   -0.03685539    0.32454220    0.47578279    0.81213562
```

We then back-transform the fifth case of principal components from the first five components.

```
@ Case5x <- Case5Y[1:5] %*% BSF
@ Case5x
           [,1]        [,2]         [,3]        [,4]        [,5]         [,6]
[1,]   -2.435065   -1.955593   -0.5789037   1.235746   1.368343   -0.9113828
```

This approximation is then compared to the fully regenerated data case and plotted in Fig. 13.5 to detect differences. Some effect is indicated in Fig. 13.5 for the forest cover variates (4 and 5).

```
@ Case5X <- Case5Y %*% t(BST)
@ Case5X
           [,1]        [,2]         [,3]        [,4]        [,5]         [,6]
[1,]   -2.434275   -1.959026   -0.5808457   1.330521   1.285380   -0.9009515@
plot(Case5X,Case5x)
```

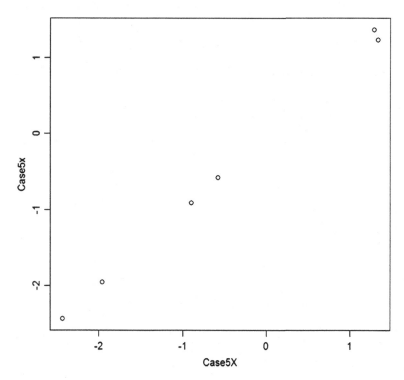

Fig. 13.5 Comparison of original values for the fifth case (*horizontal*) with values after filtering out effect of the sixth principal component

References

Afifi A, Clark V, May S (2004) Computer-aided multivariate analysis. Chapman & Hall/CRC, Boca Raton, FL

Giri N (2004) Multivariate statistical analysis. Marcel Dekker, New York

Hair J, Babin B, Anderson R (2010) Multivariate data analysis. Prentice-Hall, Upper Saddle River, NJ

Johnson R, Wichern D (2007) Applied multivariate analysis. Prenticed-Hall, Upper Saddle River, NJ

Mukhopadhyay P (2009) Multivariate statistical analysis. World Scientific, Hackensack, NJ

Rencher A (2002) Methods of multivariate analysis. Wiley-Interscience, New York

Raykov T (2008) An introduction to applied multivariate analysis. Routledge/Taylor & Francis, London

Sengupta D (2003) Linear models: an integrated approach. World Scientific, Hackensack, NJ

Timm N (2002) Applied multivariate analysis. Springer, New York

Chapter 14
Segregating Sets Along Directions of Discrimination

After general consideration of linear transformations, the previous chapter focused on decorrelation. In this chapter, attention is directed to transformations (hybridization) that can help to emphasize separation of selected groupings in the data, which falls under the scope of discriminant analysis.

As before, this topic is pursued in terms of computational context. This entails the contingents of hexagons that emerged from the clustering work in Chap. 3. Figure 14.1 shows the centroids (means) of the 11 contingents in terms of standardized scaling for the BirdSp and MamlSp variates.

```
@ Contngt <- read.table("Contingn.txt",header=T)
@ Cntr11S <- read.table("Centr11s.txt",header=T)
@ plot(Cntr11S[,1],Cntr11S[,2],xlab="BirdSpStd",ylab="MamlSpStd")
@ identify(Cntr11S[,1],Cntr11S[,2])
```

Figure 14.1 shows that contingents 4, 5, 7, and 10 are high for both birds and mammals, whereas contingents 1, 2, and 3 are low for mammals. The other four contingents (6, 8, 9, and 11) are moderate for mammals. Accordingly, we consider three groups. Group I consists of hexagons in contingents 1, 2, and 3. Group II consists of hexagons in contingents 6, 8, 9, and 11. Group III comprises hexagons in contingents 4, 5, 7, and 10. We seek a transformed view of the data that will emphasize the differences between these three groups. Our discriminant approach can only yield one fewer transformed variates than the number of groups, therefore giving us a bivariate view in this situation. We begin by segregating the groups in separate datasets that will allow plotting individual hexagons using group symbols in Fig. 14.2.

W.L. Myers and G.P. Patil, *Multivariate Methods of Representing Relations in R for Prioritization Purposes*, Environmental and Ecological Statistics 6, DOI 10.1007/978-1-4614-3122-0_14, © Springer Science+Business Media, LLC 2012

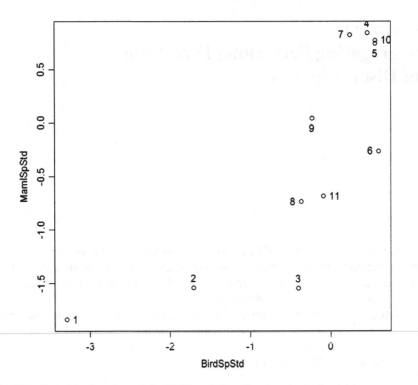

Fig. 14.1 Centroids of contingents for BirdSp and MamlSp using standardized data

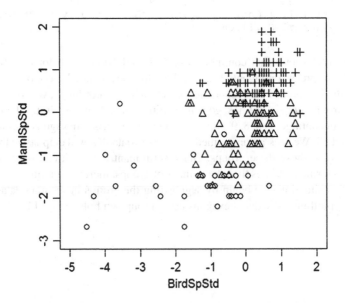

Fig. 14.2 Hexagons plotted using Group I as *circles*, Group II as *triangles*, and Group III as *crosses* with standardized data

```
@ BAMBIS <- read.table("BAMBIs.txt",header=T)
@ IhexS <- BAMBIS[Contngt$Klus11<=3,]
@ IIhexS <- BAMBIS[Contngt[,2]==6|Contngt[,2]==8|Contngt[,2]==9|
@@ Contngt[,2]==11,]
@ IIIhexS <- BAMBIS[Contngt[,2]==4|Contngt[,2]==5|Contngt[,2]==7|
@@ Contngt[,2]==10,]
@ length(IhexS[,1]) + length(IIhexS[,1]) + length(IIIhexS[,1])
[1] 211
@ plot(IhexS[,1],IhexS[,2],xlab="BirdSpStd",ylab="MamlSpStd",
@@ xlim=c(-5,2),ylim=c(-3,2),pch=1)
@ points(IIhexS[,1],IIhexS[,2],pch=2)
@ points(IIIhexS[,1],IIIhexS[,2],pch=3)
```

A propensity for progression of positioning is evident in Fig. 14.2, but is not sufficient to preclude intermingling of group constellations along the edges when seen from the perspective of standardization on the first two variates. What we seek is the possibility of transformations into a different axial perspective (or "space") whereby the segregation of groups is enhanced. Our analytical path is to find transformations that emphasize between-group variation relative to within-group variation. The first step down this path is to compute a within-group covariance matrix for each of the groups along with a collective covariance matrix for which the grouping is ignored.

Within-Groups and Collective Variation

A within-group covariance matrix is computed using only the hexagons that belong to the group. A collective covariance matrix is computed using all hexagons.

```
@ # W1 is within-group covariance matrix for group I.
@ W1 <- cov(as.data.frame(IhexS))
@ round(W1,digits=7)
              BirdSp      MamlSp     ElevSD      PctFor    Pct1FPch    Pct1OPch
BirdSp      2.0148389 -0.0167043  0.1583225  0.4364046  0.3714647 -0.6870041
MamlSp     -0.0167043  0.3068149  0.0784306  0.0870907  0.0710639 -0.0916242
ElevSD      0.1583225  0.0784306  0.1148018  0.1779256  0.1530706 -0.2059498
PctFor      0.4364046  0.0870907  0.1779256  1.2118473  1.0705360 -1.1173182
Pct1FPch    0.3714647  0.0710639  0.1530706  1.0705360  1.0271593 -0.9513863
Pct1OPch   -0.6870041 -0.0916242 -0.2059498 -1.1173182 -0.9513863  1.2830102


@ # W2 is within-group covariance matrix for group II.
@ W2 <- cov(as.data.frame(IIhexS))
@ round(W2,digits=7)
              BirdSp      MamlSp     ElevSD      PctFor    Pct1FPch    Pct1OPch
BirdSp      0.5029054  0.0949622  0.1088289 -0.0060239  0.0028413 -0.0032550
MamlSp      0.0949622  0.4027654  0.2081580  0.3054702  0.2848816 -0.3077897
ElevSD      0.1088289  0.2081580  0.6136400  0.4649986  0.4914565 -0.4344457
PctFor     -0.0060239  0.3054702  0.4649986  0.8687776  0.8384874 -0.8608308
Pct1FPch    0.0028413  0.2848816  0.4914565  0.8384874  0.8842361 -0.8463974
Pct1OPch   -0.0032550 -0.3077897 -0.4344457 -0.8608308 -0.8463974  1.2028529
```

```
@ # W3 is within-group covariance matrix for group III.
@ W3 <- cov(as.data.frame(IIIhexS))
@ round(W3,digits=7)
             BirdSp      MamlSp      ElevSD      PctFor    Pct1FPch    Pct1OPch
BirdSp    0.2449934   0.0462476  -0.0937877  -0.0499741  -0.0484493   0.0379597
MamlSp    0.0462476   0.1561237   0.0602361   0.0018023  -0.0118024   0.0074796
ElevSD   -0.0937877   0.0602361   0.9405346   0.0391293  -0.0099500   0.0126850
PctFor   -0.0499741   0.0018023   0.0391293   0.2988076   0.3073830  -0.1571698
Pct1FPch -0.0484493  -0.0118024  -0.0099500   0.3073830   0.3476463  -0.1767137
Pct1OPch  0.0379597   0.0074796   0.0126850  -0.1571698  -0.1767137   0.1150525

@ # C is collective covariance matrix.
@ C <- cov(BAMBIS)
@ C
             BirdSp      MamlSp      ElevSD      PctFor    Pct1FPch    Pct1OPch
BirdSp    1.0000000   0.5788003   0.3555759   0.2112191   0.1880800  -0.2403293
MamlSp    0.5788003   1.0000000   0.5918184   0.4829511   0.4463258  -0.4517020
ElevSD    0.3555759   0.5918184   1.0000000   0.4532556   0.4233015  -0.4025587
PctFor    0.2112191   0.4829511   0.4532556   1.0000000   0.9708868  -0.8918867
Pct1FPch  0.1880800   0.4463258   0.4233015   0.9708868   1.0000000  -0.8707050
Pct1OPch -0.2403293  -0.4517020  -0.4025587  -0.8918867  -0.8707050   1.0000000
```

The next thing is to pool the within-group covariance matrices using the degrees of freedom for the respective covariances as weights. Here, the degrees of freedom for a within-group matrix are one less than the number of cases (hexagons) in the group.

```
@ DFI <- length(IhexS[,1]) - 1
@ DFI
[1] 30
@ DFII <- length(IIhexS[,1]) -1
@ DFII
[1] 78
@ DFIII <- length(IIIhexS[,1]) -1
@ DFIII
[1] 100
@ DFI + DFII + DFIII
[1] 208
@ DFdiv <- 1/208
@ W <- DFI * W1 + DFII * W2 + DFIII * W3
@ W <- W * DFdiv
@ round(W,digits=7)
             BirdSp      MamlSp      ElevSD      PctFor    Pct1FPch    Pct1OPch
BirdSp    0.5969766   0.0554360   0.0185556   0.0366580   0.0313492  -0.0820579
MamlSp    0.0554360   0.2703486   0.1183310   0.1279790   0.1114060  -0.1250402
ElevSD    0.0185556   0.1183310   0.6988531   0.2188489   0.2015900  -0.1865229
PctFor    0.0366580   0.1279790   0.2188489   0.6442348   0.6166173  -0.5595256
Pct1FPch  0.0313492   0.1114060   0.2015900   0.6166173   0.6468742  -0.5395767
Pct1OPch -0.0820579  -0.1250402  -0.1865229  -0.5595256  -0.5395767   0.6914331
```

Between-Groups Variation

Between-groups variation is computed as the weighted difference between the collective variation and the pooled within-groups variation, then treating this difference as having degrees of freedom that is one less than the number of groups.

```
@ PDF <- DFI + DFII + DFIII
@ B <- 210 * C - PDF * W
@ B <- B * 0.5
@ round(B,digits=7)
          BirdSp    MamlSp    ElevSD    PctFor   Pct1FPch  Pct1OPch
BirdSp    42.91443  55.00870  35.40569  18.36558  16.48809 -16.70056
MamlSp    55.00870  76.88374  49.83450  37.40005  35.27799 -34.42453
ElevSD    35.40569  49.83450  32.31928  24.83154  23.48129 -22.87028
PctFor    18.36558  37.40005  24.83154  37.99958  37.81491 -35.45744
Pct1FPch  16.48809  35.27799  23.48129  37.81491  37.72509 -35.30805
Pct1OPch -16.70056 -34.42453 -22.87028 -35.45744 -35.30805  33.09096
```

Formulation and Computation

The calculus approach to optimization leads to the following as a precursor for eigenvector analysis:

$$\mathbf{BH_K} = \mathbf{WH_K}\lambda_k$$

where $\mathbf{B}$ is the between-groups variation matrix, $\mathbf{W}$ is the (pooled) within-groups variation matrix, $\mathbf{H_K}$ is a transformation vector, and λ_k a corresponding eigenvalue.

Developing this in the more obvious way gives:

$$\mathbf{W^{-1}BH_K} = \mathbf{W^{-1}WH_K}\lambda_k$$

$$\mathbf{W^{-1}BH_K} = \mathbf{H_K}\lambda_k$$

This then entails computing eigenvalues and eigenvectors of the $\mathbf{W^{-1}B}$ product matrix, which is not a symmetric matrix. However, computing eigenvectors of an asymmetric matrix is problematic. Therefore, it is appropriate to use a more complicated alternate development that leads to finding eigenvalues and eigenvectors of a symmetric matrix.

The alternate development relies on Cholesky decomposition of the symmetric $\mathbf{W}$ matrix. To this end, let $\mathbf{L}$ be the upper-triangular result produced by the chol() function in $\mathbf{R}$ when applied to the $\mathbf{W}$ matrix:

```
L<- chol(W)
```

An upper-triangular matrix has only zero elements below the diagonal, and a lower-triangular matrix has only zero elements above the diagonal. The decomposition has the property that $\mathbf{L'L = W}$. Then, the alternate development proceeds as follows, where we note that the inverse of a transpose is the transpose of the inverse.

$$\mathbf{BH}_K = \mathbf{WH}_K \lambda_k$$

$$\mathbf{BH}_K = \mathbf{L'LH}_K \lambda_k$$

$$(\mathbf{L'})^{-1} \mathbf{BH}_K = (\mathbf{L'})^{-1} \mathbf{L'LH}_K \lambda_k$$

$$(\mathbf{L'})^{-1} \mathbf{BH}_K = \mathbf{LH}_K \lambda_k$$

$$(\mathbf{L'})^{-1} \mathbf{BL}^{-1}\mathbf{LH}_K = \mathbf{LH}_K \lambda_k$$

$$(\mathbf{L}^{-1})' \mathbf{BL}^{-1} (\mathbf{LH}_K) = (\mathbf{LH}_K) \lambda_k$$

Now, let $\mathbf{Q} = \mathbf{L}^{-1}$ and $\mathbf{V} = \mathbf{LH}_K$. Then, we have

$$(\mathbf{Q'BQ})\mathbf{V} = \mathbf{V}\lambda_k$$

which calls for finding λ_k and $\mathbf{V}$ as eigenvalue and eigenvector, respectively of $\mathbf{Q'BQ}$. Since $\mathbf{V} = \mathbf{LH}_K$ we obtain $\mathbf{H}_K = \mathbf{L}^{-1}\mathbf{V} = \mathbf{QV}$. Any eigenvector corresponding to an eigenvalue that is effectively zero is meaningless and should not be used.

Accordingly, $\mathbf{L}$ and $\mathbf{Q}$ are computed, and then $\mathbf{Q'BQ}$ is obtained as $\mathbf{A}$.

```
@ L <- chol(W)
@ Q <- solve(L)
@ A <- t(Q) %*% B
@ A <- A %*% Q
@ round(A,digits=7)
              BirdSp      MamlSp     ElevSD       PctFor    Pct1FPch    Pct1OPch
BirdSp     71.886292  128.234574  18.7242489  -19.6253574   7.7764172  13.5775648
MamlSp    128.234574  252.780014  37.3816783   -7.4563759  22.2968901  20.7744178
ElevSD     18.724249   37.381678   5.5364719   -0.5476946   3.4211358   2.9657200
PctFor    -19.625357   -7.456376  -0.5476946   36.9510127   7.5374891  -7.6580931
Pct1FPch    7.776417   22.296890   3.4211358    7.5374891   3.7951916   0.2605424
Pct1OPch   13.577565   20.774418   2.9657200   -7.6580931   0.2605424   3.0586627
```

An extraction of characteristic roots and vectors is performed on $\mathbf{A}$, with the eigenvectors designated as $\mathbf{V}$. Only the first two eigenvalues are nonzero, so only the first two eigenvectors will be retained at the end of the process.

```
@ Egns <- eigen(A)
@ summary(Egns)
        Length Class  Mode
values    6      -none- numeric
vectors  36      -none- numeric
@ round(Egns$values,digits=6)
[1] 329.1828  44.8248    0.0000    0.0000    0.0000    0.0000
@ V <- Egns$vectors
@ V
             [,1]          [,2]          [,3]          [,4]          [,5]          [,6]
[1,] -0.45489776  0.28992579  0.00000000  0.84202795  0.00000000  0.00000000
[2,] -0.87332455 -0.19552455 -0.05610592 -0.40448274 -0.16956549  0.05973070
[3,] -0.12873365 -0.04254529 -0.28592516 -0.05489803  0.94667496  0.02563337
[4,]  0.05326434 -0.89638620  0.10603450  0.33741791  0.01146750  0.26158944
[5,] -0.07089669 -0.21852910  0.31520181  0.03694233  0.10263810 -0.91431242
[6,] -0.07704849  0.15697103  0.89694116 -0.09567276  0.25374786  0.30228950
```

The modal matrix of eigenvectors is shown to be orthogonal as expected from the symmetry of its parent matrix.

```
@ round((t(V)  %*%  V),digits=6)
     [,1] [,2] [,3] [,4] [,5] [,6]
[1,]    1    0    0    0    0    0
[2,]    0    1    0    0    0    0
[3,]    0    0    1    0    0    0
[4,]    0    0    0    1    0    0
[5,]    0    0    0    0    1    0
[6,]    0    0    0    0    0    1
```

Finally, the transformation (hybridization) vectors **H** are computed by multiplying eigenvectors by the **Q** matrix. The last four columns of the matrix are then discarded due to their meaningless nature as reflected in the degenerate eigenvalues.

```
@ H <- Q %*% V
@ H
              [,1]          [,2]          [,3]          [,4]          [,5]          [,6]
BirdSp   -0.4491036  0.46052854  0.1700959  1.1358817  0.08895470  0.02648308
MamlSp   -1.6723994  0.05822333  0.1482423 -0.9235456 -0.80677006 -0.15684526
ElevSD   -0.1785785  0.24277225 -0.4041168 -0.1800664  1.16991993 -0.09405718
PctFor    0.2282055 -0.05152276  0.4137363  0.1410261  0.03686188  4.61621458
Pct1FPch -0.3137189 -0.89261748  1.4993046  0.1378610  0.48098812 -3.80149313
Pct1OPch -0.1721331  0.35068699  2.0038449 -0.2137413  0.56689487  0.67534114
@ H <- H[,1:2]
@ H
              [,1]          [,2]
BirdSp   -0.4491036  0.46052854
MamlSp   -1.6723994  0.05822333
ElevSD   -0.1785785  0.24277225
PctFor    0.2282055 -0.05152276
Pct1FPch -0.3137189 -0.89261748
Pct1OPch -0.1721331  0.35068699
```

A point of particular interest is that the transformation is scaled so that $\mathbf{H'WH = I}$ which will be explored subsequently relative to Mahalanobis (generalized) distance.

```
@ round((t(H) %*% W %*% H),digits=6)
     [,1] [,2]
[1,]    1    0
[2,]    0    1
```

Canonical Variates

The transformation is applied to the data (which were previously standardized) to obtain what can be called *canonical variates* or *discriminant axes*. Usage of standardized data as a starting point was simply a matter of choice in the present situation. Here, we designate the canonical variates as **G** by virtue of the relation to Mahalanobis generalized distance (Digby and Kempton 1987), which has yet to be explored here.

The hexagon data for each of the groups will be transformed separately for convenience in plotting and subsequent comparison. Since the hexagon data are as a data frame whereas the transformations are matrix operations, the operands must recast appropriately.

```
@ IhexG <- as.matrix(IhexS) %*% H
@ IhexG <- as.data.frame(IhexG)
@ summary(IhexG)
          V1                    V2
 Min.    :1.343    Min.    :-3.23543
 1st Qu.:2.760     1st Qu.:-1.95884
 Median :3.310     Median :-0.60279
 Mean    :3.473    Mean    :-0.90800
 3rd Qu.:3.996     3rd Qu.: 0.02008
 Max.    :6.377    Max.    : 1.17315


@ IIhexG <- as.matrix(IIhexS) %*% H
@ IIhexG <- as.data.frame(IIhexG)
@ summary(IIhexG)
          V1                    V2
 Min.    :-1.7088    Min.    :-1.9675
 1st Qu.:-0.2997     1st Qu.:-0.3297
 Median : 0.4938     Median : 0.9795
 Mean    : 0.6519    Mean    : 0.8075
 3rd Qu.: 1.3411     3rd Qu.: 1.5174
 Max.    : 3.5025    Max.    : 2.9685


@ IIIhexG <- as.matrix(IIIhexS) %*% H
@ IIIhexG <- as.data.frame(IIIhexG)
@ summary(IIIhexG)
          V1                    V2
 Min.    :-3.4792    Min.    :-1.72612
 1st Qu.:-2.0489     1st Qu.:-0.92832
 Median :-1.5816     Median :-0.44389
 Mean    :-1.5759     Mean    :-0.35291
 3rd Qu.:-1.0585     3rd Qu.: 0.05937
 Max.    :-0.1288     Max.    : 1.75290
```

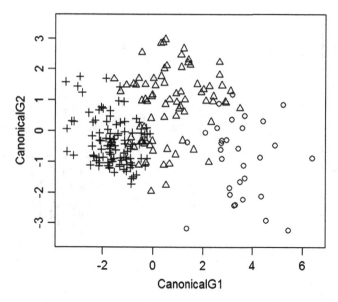

Fig. 14.3 Hexagons plotted using Group I as *circles*, Group II as *triangles*, and Group III as *crosses* with canonical (G) variates

We are now prepared to plot the counterpart of Fig. 14.2 using canonical variates instead of standardized variates to obtain Fig. 14.3.

```
@ plot(IhexG[,1],IhexG[,2],xlab="CanonicalG1",ylab="CanonicalG2",
@@ xlim=c(-3.5,6.5),ylim=c(-3.5,3.5),pch=1)
@ points(IIhexG[,1],IIhexG[,2],pch=2)
@ points(IIIhexG[,1],IIIhexG[,2],pch=3)
```

Comparing Fig. 14.3 to Fig. 14.2 we again observe a logical axis reversal, this time for the first (G1) canonical axis which has Group I on the high end instead of the low end. Again, the signs on the axes arising from eigen analysis are essentially arbitrary, and there is nothing to inhibit changing the sense of sign. This could be done either directly in the **H** matrix or within the transformed data frames, but we arbitrarily choose the latter.

The axis adjustment is done as follows, and the groups are then replotted on the adjusted canonical axes in Fig. 14.4.

```
@ IhexG[,1] <- IhexG[,1] * -1.0
@ summary(IhexG)
        V1                 V2
 Min.    :-6.377   Min.    :-3.23543
 1st Qu.:-3.996    1st Qu.:-1.95884
 Median :-3.310    Median :-0.60279
 Mean    :-3.473   Mean    :-0.90800
 3rd Qu.:-2.760    3rd Qu.: 0.02008
 Max.    :-1.343   Max.     : 1.17315
@ IIhexG[,1] <- IIhexG[,1] * -1.0
@ summary(IIhexG)
        V1                 V2
 Min.    :-3.5025   Min.    :-1.9675
 1st Qu.:-1.3411    1st Qu.:-0.3297
```

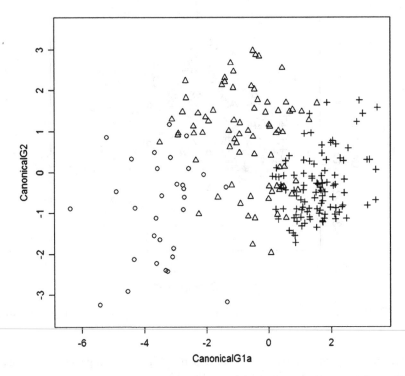

Fig. 14.4 Hexagons plotted using Group I as *circles*, Group II as *triangles*, and Group III as *crosses* with sign-adjusted canonical variates

```
Median :-0.4938    Median : 0.9795
Mean   :-0.6519    Mean    : 0.8075
3rd Qu.: 0.2997    3rd Qu.: 1.5174
Max.   : 1.7088    Max.    : 2.9685
@ IIIhexG[,1] <- IIIhexG[,1] * -1.0
@ summary(IIIhexG)
          V1                 V2
Min.   :0.1288     Min.    :-1.72612
1st Qu.:1.0585     1st Qu.:-0.92832
Median :1.5816     Median :-0.44389
Mean   :1.5759     Mean    :-0.35291
3rd Qu.:2.0489     3rd Qu.: 0.05937
Max.   :3.4792     Max.    : 1.75290
@ plot(IhexG[,1],IhexG[,2],xlab="CanonicalG1a",ylab="CanonicalG2",
@@ xlim=c(-6.5,3.5),ylim=c(-3.5,3.5),pch=1)
@ points(IIhexG[,1],IIhexG[,2],pch=2)
@ points(IIIhexG[,1],IIIhexG[,2],pch=3)
```

In Fig. 14.4, axis 1 has the primary gradient of difference between the groups and axis 2 has emphasis on sorting out Group II. Another way of summarizing the plot is that the upper-left to lower-right diagonal separates Group I from the other two groups, and Group II separates from Group III across the lower-left to upper-right diagonal.

Canonical (discriminant) axes serve to maximum advantage when the within-group covariance matrices are essentially the same. There are some differences in this regard for the hexagons, which tends to impede the separability of group constellations somewhat.

Mahalanobis Generalized Distance

It was observed above that $\mathbf{H'WH} = \mathbf{I}$, from which we obtain:

$$\mathbf{H'WH} = \mathbf{I}$$

$$\left(\mathbf{H'}\right)^{-1}\mathbf{H'WH} = \left(\mathbf{H'}\right)^{-1}\mathbf{I}$$

$$\mathbf{WH} = \left(\mathbf{H'}\right)^{-1}$$

$$\mathbf{WHH}^{-1} = \left(\mathbf{H'}\right)^{-1}\mathbf{H}^{-1} = \left(\mathbf{HH'}\right)^{-1}$$

$$\mathbf{W} = \left(\mathbf{HH'}\right)^{-1}$$

$$\mathbf{W}^{-1} = \mathbf{HH'}$$

Now, consider the distance between two points in data space ($\mathbf{X}_1$ and $\mathbf{X}_2$) after transformation into canonical space:

$$\mathbf{G}_1 = \mathbf{X}_1\mathbf{H} \text{ and } \mathbf{G}_2 = \mathbf{X}_2\mathbf{H}$$

$$\mathbf{D}^2 = \left(\mathbf{G}_1 - \mathbf{G}_2\right)\left(\mathbf{G}_1 - \mathbf{G}_2\right)'$$

$$\mathbf{D}^2 = \left(\mathbf{X}_1\mathbf{H} - \mathbf{X}_2\mathbf{H}\right)\left(\mathbf{X}_1\mathbf{H} - \mathbf{X}_2\mathbf{H}\right)'$$

$$\mathbf{D}^2 = \left(\mathbf{X}_1 - \mathbf{X}_2\right)\mathbf{H}\left[\left(\mathbf{X}_1 - \mathbf{X}_2\right)\mathbf{H}\right]'$$

$$\mathbf{D}^2 = \left(\mathbf{X}_1 - \mathbf{X}_2\right)\mathbf{HH'}\left(\mathbf{X}_1 - \mathbf{X}_2\right)$$

$$\mathbf{D}^2 = \left(\mathbf{X}_1 - \mathbf{X}_2\right)\mathbf{W}^{-1}\left(\mathbf{X}_1 - \mathbf{X}_2\right)$$

This latter is termed (squared) *Mahalanobis distance* or *generalized distance*. Thus, Mahalanobis distance computed from data matrices corresponds to Euclidean distance computed in canonical variate (or discriminant) space. This shows that Mahalanobis distance gives direct computation of distance in canonical variate space without first transforming the data.

Special Spaces

The principal axis and canonical axis work in Part III exemplify transformations of data into special coordinate spaces that confer particular analytical advantages. These two types of transformations fall within a general class of *linear transformations* (hybridizations) that involve axial rotation and rescaling. If we again use $\mathbf{X}^{n \times p}$ as the notation for a data matrix consisting of n cases with p variates, such transformations can be represented as:

$$\mathbf{Y}^{n \times q} = (\mathbf{X}^{n \times p}) \times (\mathbf{H}^{p \times q})$$

where $\mathbf{H}^{p \times q}$ is a transformation (hybridization) matrix having p rows and q columns in which each column generates a transformed variate (axis) as a linear combination of the original p variates with the element in a particular row being the weight given to the corresponding original variate in forming the transformed variate as a weighted composite (summation) of the original variates. The transformation will be reversible (invertible) only if $q = p$ and $\mathbf{H}$ is nonsingular.

The transformation entails simple axial rotations if the columns of $\mathbf{H}$ are normalized (length = 1.0); otherwise, there is some rescaling (expansion or contraction) along with rotation. In the latter case, the transformation can be expressed as a product:

$$\mathbf{H}^{p \times q} = \left(\mathbf{A}^{p \times q}\right) \times \left(\mathbf{M}^{q \times q}\right)$$

where the $\mathbf{A}$ matrix has the angular rotation information expressed as direction cosines, with $\mathbf{A}$ being obtained by normalizing the columns of $\mathbf{H}$. $\mathbf{M}$ is a diagonal matrix of multipliers that rescale the respective axes after rotation, wherein the multiplicative scaling factors are the reciprocals of the normalizing factors for obtaining $\mathbf{A}$ from $\mathbf{H}$.

There are other interesting (multivariate) transformations in this class which we have not considered, such as those from canonical correlation analysis which seeks paired linear transformations that emphasize the relationships among two sets of variables. Facilities for this and many other "special space" analyses are available without cost from the CRAN library of contributed **R** analyses which includes more than 2,000 contributed packages. Canonical correlation analysis is available in the *CCA* package among others. The foregoing treatment of matrix transformations in **R** should provide a foundation for exploring such facilities (Bloomfield 2009).

There are also major methods of recasting data in various interesting coordinate systems that do not fall within the general class of linear transformations. The principal coordinate analysis in Part II, Chap. 5 is one such approach. Of related interest to the approaches we have presented is a large class of *ordination* methods that are extensively used by ecologists (McCune and Grace 2002; Leps 2003; Soetaert and Herman 2009; Wildi 2010), and can be explored through the ***vegan*** package in the CRAN library. A tool of interest in conjunction with cross-tabulations is *correspondence analysis* (Greenacre and Blasius 2006) which provides a graphic method of exploring relationships between variables in a contingency table. The ***anacor*** package in the CRAN library provides a point of departure in this regard.

References

Bloomfield V (2009) Computer simulation and data analysis in molecular biology and biophysics: an introduction using R. Springer, New York

Digby P, Kempton R (1987) Multivariate analysis of ecological communities. Chapman & Hall, New York

Greenacre M, Blasius J (2006) Multiple correspondence analysis and related methods. Chapman & Hall/CRC, Boca Raton, FL

Leps J (2003) Multivariate analysis of ecological data using CANOCO. Cambridge University Press, Cambridge, UK

McCune B, Grace J (2002) Analysis of ecological communities. MjM Software Design, Gleneden Beach, OR

Soetaert K, Herman P (2009) A practical guide to ecological modeling: using R as a simulation platform. Springer, Dordrecht

Wildi O (2010) Data analysis in vegetation ecology. Wiley-Blackwell, Chichester

Appendix 1
Printout of BAMBI.txt File of Pennsylvania Hexagon Data

HexNo	BirdSp	MamlSp	ElevSD	PctFor	Pct1FPch	Pct1OPch
1714	55	34	11	35.4	35.4	64.6
1827	58	37	32	84.3	84.0	7.4
1828	116	37	27	50.3	47.5	27.2
1829	96	34	17	25.3	20.3	60.3
1941	86	37	51	100.0	100.0	0.0
1942	118	39	35	74.2	74.1	12.3
1943	110	36	23	64.1	61.4	11.4
1944	120	37	43	69.0	68.6	16.0
2053	99	47	88	96.7	96.7	2.5
2054	125	47	95	94.0	94.0	1.2
2055	132	45	78	93.8	93.7	4.2
2056	124	42	75	50.2	46.4	29.6
2057	123	39	46	67.1	56.3	24.0
2058	118	37	41	81.2	77.0	5.2
2059	115	37	43	85.7	85.7	2.1
2060	107	38	26	95.1	95.1	1.1
2061	96	37	31	88.2	84.2	5.0
2169	114	48	49	92.0	92.0	8.0
2170	139	49	66	96.9	96.9	1.8
2171	132	50	104	97.5	97.5	0.9
2172	141	48	138	69.7	69.5	12.7
2173	128	42	66	56.2	50.7	29.2
2174	115	40	52	45.3	24.6	52.8
2175	117	40	69	81.6	81.3	8.0
2176	118	39	39	67.6	67.0	14.7
2177	119	38	32	37.6	36.0	43.5
2178	106	38	35	59.0	30.1	33.4
2286	120	49	96	99.2	99.2	0.5
2287	129	49	57	91.0	90.2	6.0
2288	130	50	75	91.8	91.3	2.1
2289	134	50	45	95.2	94.2	2.8
2290	137	49	95	93.4	93.1	1.7
2291	145	45	83	74.2	71.6	11.5
2292	141	46	78	49.9	46.0	33.1

(continued)

W.L. Myers and G.P. Patil, *Multivariate Methods of Representing Relations
in R for Prioritization Purposes*, Environmental and Ecological Statistics 6,
DOI 10.1007/978-1-4614-3122-0, © Springer Science+Business Media, LLC 2012

(continued)

HexNo	BirdSp	MamlSp	ElevSD	PctFor	Pct1FPch	Pct1OPch
2293	132	38	56	54.6	43.8	26.4
2294	103	39	15	11.9	8.2	46.4
2295	125	40	57	59.5	58.1	8.9
2296	84	38	28	47.2	14.1	35.6
2404	104	48	181	99.5	99.5	0.2
2405	129	51	70	96.7	96.7	0.8
2406	125	49	88	79.7	79.7	9.5
2407	131	48	104	58.4	37.6	36.8
2408	136	50	128	78.7	68.3	12.3
2409	130	45	89	80.8	80.8	11.2
2410	128	43	105	85.4	85.2	4.0
2411	132	44	81	53.7	48.1	35.5
2412	123	40	33	35.1	29.0	46.5
2413	117	40	36	39.1	36.9	49.2
2414	108	38	41	51.0	27.8	36.5
2415	67	38	23	41.2	18.5	29.0
2524	103	48	187	94.1	77.8	2.1
2525	123	48	55	87.5	87.4	3.1
2526	143	49	73	80.7	79.5	3.6
2527	135	49	120	88.6	88.4	4.1
2528	138	47	67	80.0	79.6	2.3
2529	133	45	103	74.3	70.5	7.6
2530	123	45	83	82.5	81.5	9.4
2531	134	45	111	81.2	77.4	17.1
2532	128	44	38	59.7	51.1	23.3
2533	115	39	36	63.4	60.7	26.1
2534	115	39	36	38.3	18.6	49.7
2645	115	48	205	91.9	91.0	2.6
2646	132	48	55	89.1	88.7	1.9
2647	133	48	135	95.7	95.6	0.9
2648	129	52	126	98.5	98.4	0.5
2649	127	47	65	66.0	64.8	8.5
2650	120	46	56	69.8	66.4	5.5
2651	121	46	62	62.5	60.8	11.1
2652	129	45	70	80.1	72.6	5.1
2653	132	43	57	62.3	45.1	32.4
2654	125	42	75	70.5	70.2	8.7
2655	119	41	107	80.5	78.4	7.3
2767	114	48	72	94.9	94.8	1.2
2768	130	48	83	76.8	73.7	8.8
2769	129	49	78	99.2	99.2	0.3
2770	131	50	119	83.1	82.5	7.1
2771	135	47	81	48.9	46.4	30.4
2772	130	46	54	47.5	23.9	22.3
2773	122	46	101	76.6	74.4	6.7
2774	126	46	80	77.1	75.3	10.3
2775	140	42	110	53.4	46.8	32.0
2776	134	43	121	51.2	46.9	46.2
2777	117	41	85	27.7	19.4	68.4
2890	106	47	87	81.2	78.4	8.7
2891	126	49	114	83.2	83.0	1.6
2892	130	47	108	95.6	95.6	1.2
2893	130	50	118	70.0	69.2	9.5
2894	126	47	114	89.4	89.3	4.5
2895	135	47	130	84.7	84.7	6.3
2896	123	49	114	75.4	70.9	6.6

(continued)

(continued)

HexNo	BirdSp	MamlSp	ElevSD	PctFor	Pct1FPch	Pct1OPch
2897	129	48	114	83.2	82.6	8.8
2898	128	47	115	75.7	75.4	10.7
2899	126	44	127	58.3	52.1	34.1
2900	116	42	99	53.7	48.3	27.7
3014	129	47	72	89.6	89.6	2.7
3015	134	48	79	87.7	87.7	2.1
3016	128	49	80	86.9	86.6	5.6
3017	131	48	132	91.3	89.0	4.7
3018	132	48	123	71.9	69.1	16.5
3019	133	53	102	59.3	37.2	23.4
3020	136	51	117	68.7	49.1	16.7
3021	122	46	110	89.8	89.8	2.0
3022	128	47	123	87.0	85.8	4.4
3023	118	46	110	74.4	73.7	5.1
3024	111	44	80	80.8	70.4	5.9
3139	129	47	78	82.7	73.7	9.7
3140	137	49	90	87.4	87.2	7.9
3141	128	49	97	100.0	100.0	0.0
3142	124	49	124	98.9	98.9	0.5
3143	132	50	118	91.0	90.9	2.8
3144	145	51	99	67.4	38.1	17.5
3145	131	50	94	67.4	64.3	11.1
3146	128	48	103	68.8	49.1	23.1
3147	129	48	94	69.7	67.4	13.9
3148	120	47	92	78.1	77.0	7.8
3149	104	45	102	96.6	96.6	1.3
3265	135	49	69	82.7	78.8	8.3
3266	137	50	76	96.2	96.2	2.5
3267	127	50	94	99.5	99.5	0.5
3268	127	50	117	99.2	99.2	0.5
3269	132	49	77	72.0	65.1	16.3
3270	123	49	111	77.2	76.0	6.6
3271	129	49	144	70.6	66.8	21.1
3272	120	48	150	78.0	65.0	9.5
3273	139	48	166	71.3	45.4	15.8
3274	132	48	138	89.0	87.1	3.8
3275	117	45	156	76.4	72.6	7.6
3391	98	46	66	75.4	71.2	13.3
3392	130	49	61	85.8	85.7	4.0
3393	137	48	77	97.4	97.4	0.7
3394	126	48	98	99.0	99.0	0.7
3395	122	48	87	96.2	96.1	1.1
3396	116	48	78	68.8	67.7	7.3
3397	120	47	55	68.6	66.8	7.7
3398	115	49	49	57.4	44.6	18.0
3399	126	49	102	67.7	53.5	16.8
3400	144	51	65	53.6	46.1	26.2
3401	135	52	82	67.6	66.1	7.9
3402	69	46	68	99.4	99.4	0.6
3519	99	46	69	87.1	65.6	4.0
3520	138	48	74	83.2	81.8	4.9
3521	131	49	68	99.8	99.8	0.2
3522	129	49	61	79.7	78.0	9.0
3523	138	49	63	70.6	59.8	25.5
3524	128	48	61	60.3	41.2	22.7

(continued)

(continued)

HexNo	BirdSp	MamlSp	ElevSD	PctFor	Pct1FPch	Pct1OPch
3525	117	48	52	48.1	18.9	37.4
3526	129	49	92	72.8	69.4	8.4
3527	134	52	142	84.6	84.1	7.9
3528	133	52	114	74.3	70.6	8.7
3529	129	53	97	90.0	90.0	1.8
3648	118	47	77	93.4	88.1	5.7
3649	137	47	54	94.2	94.2	2.5
3650	130	49	45	90.3	90.2	4.3
3651	130	48	49	89.9	89.8	5.1
3652	126	47	43	62.2	48.6	8.7
3653	116	47	40	40.1	30.4	32.9
3654	118	45	32	42.8	15.8	53.5
3655	115	46	33	48.9	45.6	33.7
3656	127	45	83	30.7	18.7	66.5
3657	126	45	116	60.4	49.4	23.2
3658	130	47	146	66.3	49.2	30.9
3778	127	47	87	98.9	98.8	0.7
3779	122	47	68	97.0	97.0	0.7
3780	119	48	45	99.1	99.1	0.8
3781	128	46	38	89.5	89.5	3.6
3782	123	47	39	41.9	26.4	42.6
3783	126	43	51	47.1	34.3	19.0
3784	127	43	45	54.9	45.5	14.6
3785	101	40	35	28.2	6.3	70.5
3786	121	40	40	48.6	27.1	23.0
3787	113	39	33	58.8	53.0	17.5
3788	109	39	40	91.0	90.6	4.0
3909	124	46	69	70.2	64.8	11.2
3910	129	47	61	94.7	93.0	1.0
3911	133	48	49	95.2	95.1	2.7
3912	130	46	33	69.9	69.4	11.3
3913	127	44	47	49.6	37.9	21.2
3914	111	42	27	24.3	7.9	74.9
3915	116	42	38	27.0	5.5	67.6
3916	112	39	39	16.0	2.2	65.0
3917	115	39	27	54.5	29.2	44.3
3918	109	39	34	95.4	94.8	2.4
3919	102	39	34	98.1	98.1	1.9
4041	127	46	39	63.6	55.8	12.7
4042	132	47	38	75.6	73.7	5.9
4043	129	48	47	80.3	79.7	2.0
4044	130	46	43	70.1	68.2	18.3
4045	142	43	24	30.1	10.0	64.5
4046	118	42	32	19.0	2.3	80.4
4047	114	42	41	38.0	10.9	35.2
4048	110	40	26	38.4	26.8	56.1
4049	109	38	31	82.8	82.6	4.7
4050	104	39	37	100.0	100.0	0.0
4173	109	43	67	43.7	27.3	35.2
4174	133	44	45	45.4	13.3	33.0

(continued)

(continued)

HexNo	BirdSp	MamlSp	ElevSD	PctFor	Pct1FPch	Pct1OPch
4175	142	45	38	52.0	43.6	16.3
4176	133	45	36	52.3	45.8	76.8
4177	128	43	30	22.9	5.2	85.5
4178	127	42	42	14.0	2.6	48.2
4179	115	42	37	30.8	7.4	12.3
4180	100	41	39	50.0	37.2	1.1
4306	75	40	20	8.6	7.2	84.7
4307	130	43	98	32.5	8.5	57.2
4308	128	44	40	45.4	11.2	44.8
4309	143	44	33	47.8	33.4	23.8
4310	120	43	37	37.5	22.3	31.8
4311	109	43	31	23.9	8.7	73.0
4312	63	41	27	17.6	17.6	76.1
4442	105	41	33	42.6	34.2	27.5
4443	126	43	42	54.0	32.8	36.6
4444	113	43	16	66.5	57.9	26.2

Appendix 2
R~Workshop I—Getting Started with R

R is open-source software made available under the auspices of the R Foundation without cost for unlimited usage. It is a statistical analysis system and a computational + graphics programming language. It has a commercial counterpart called S-Plus distributed by Insightful Corporation. Both are based on the **S** language, which was developed at Bell Laboratories. There are also a large number of extensions to **R** for special purposes that have been contributed by users and are freely available. **R** simplifies conventional statistical analyses, while also permitting customized approaches to be set up and applied. Although **R** is available for several types of computers, this workshop assumes that you will be using a PC running a Windows© operating system.

Obtaining R

A good place to start in obtaining **R** is at the Web site http://www.r-project.org for the Foundation, which has links to download and other sites of interest—particularly, the CRAN Web site cran.r-project.org the "Comprehensive R Archive Network". A binary setup module for installation on a Windows PC can be downloaded along with documentation. Proceed to download and unzip the files as necessary.

Installing R

Installation of **R** is accomplished by double-clicking the *.exe* for installation setup. The main part of the name for this file consists of the version designation. You will need administrative privileges on the computer to perform the installation, but you will not need such privileges to run the software after it is installed. The option to create an icon on the desktop should be accepted, since it will be desirable to specify the startup folder as a property of the icon when you launch it.

Starting and Stopping R

Before launching **R**, create a working folder near the root of a disk so that it does not have a long path. Launch **R** either from an icon or the program menu. When the **R** desktop appears, go to the File menu, choose "Change dir…" and navigate to the working folder. All files in the working folder will be readable by **R** without specifying a path. To quit R, enter q() at the > R prompt, or go to the File menu and choose "Exit".

R as a Calculator

If you type in 2+2 and press ENTER, the response from **R** will be 4
  The calculator operators in **R** are + − * / ^ (power)

%/% (integer division)
%% (integer remainder)

  Other algebraic operators are functions having a function name and the inputs enclosed in parentheses, with sqrt() and log10() being examples.

R Help

Type either ?help or help() to see how help works in **R**.
  To get help with an **R** command, you put the name of the command in the help() parentheses, or put a question mark before the name of the command without any parentheses.
  Type in list.files() or dir() to get a listing of the files in the working folder.
  To try finding an **R** facility for some purpose, use help.search ("keyword") where the keyword is some keyword for the topic. The keyword must be enclosed in quotes.
  If you are connected to the internet, you can start a Web help with help.start ().

R Objects

R works with objects having names that consist of letters and digits with periods as optional separators like July10.data.2007 as an example. Object names for **R** are case sensitive, so a name with a capital is different from one in lower case. Since **R** has most of its operators named with lower-case, it is a good idea to start the names of your objects with a capital letter so that you do not inadvertently mess things up.

There are several different kinds of objects in **R**, and an object has properties depending on its kind. Among the several kinds of objects are

- A container for a unitary value (actually a single-valued vector);
- A vector containing a set of values with the same properties in a specified order;
- A matrix containing a row and column layout of values with the same properties;
- A data frame as a "cases-by-variates" table with row cases and column variates;
- A list as a container for aggregating different kinds of objects;
- A statistical model;
- A function to do operations.

Properties of an object indicate the type(s) of values that it contains, such as numeric, categorical (factors with levels), logical (True, False, NA), or names. The type can be changed by coercion, as for example as.factor() for changing numeric codes into categorical factors. A missing value should be coded as NA for not available.

The relational operators among objects are

==	equal
!=	not equal
<	less than
>	greater than
<=	less than or equal
>=	greater than or equal
&	and
|	or
!	not
is.na()	missing value
!is.na()	not a missing value

Content is assigned to objects with the <– two-character symbol of less than followed immediately by a minus sign. It can be considered as "put into" the object on the left what is specified on the right.

Components are indexed in square brackets, as for ht[5] for the fifth component of a vector having ht as its name. A sequence is indicated by a colon, as in [2:6] for 2 through 6. An omitted index extracts the entire range of the index, as in MatrxA[,3] to get column 3.

The vector of values for a variable as a column component of a data frame is extracted by the $ selector, as in FrameName$VarName where each column is separately named.

Data Entry

The simplest way to enter a short set of values into a vector is with the c() concatenation command, as for example

> VecA <- c(2,6,9,12,20)
> VecA
[1] 2 6 9 12 20

As can be seen, entering the name of the vector by itself gives the values comprising the vector. The commands and output preceding this paragraph were taken by "cut and paste" from the R window, which is a reasonable way to save R output without all of the dialog you may not want.

The typical mode of entering statistical data, however, will be as a data frame in the form of a table. The dataset to be used here for illustration is from Altman 1991. Practical statistics for medical research (Exercise 12.5, 10.1). Chapman & Hall.

It has been incorporated in the ISwR package for R by Dalgaard 2002. Introductory statistics with R. Springer.

There are 32 rows and 4 columns, with the columns being as follows

Age of subject (years)
Sex, with F=1, M=2
Height of subject (cm)
Total lung capacity (l) of subject prior to organ transplant.

A listing of the data follows:

age	sex	ht	tlc
35	1	149	3.40
11	1	138	3.41
12	2	148	3.80
16	1	156	3.90
32	1	152	4.00
16	1	157	4.10
14	1	165	4.46
16	2	152	4.55
35	1	177	4.83
33	1	158	5.10
40	1	166	5.44
28	1	165	5.50
23	1	160	5.73
52	2	178	5.77
46	1	169	5.80
29	2	173	6.00
30	1	172	6.30
21	1	163	6.55

```
21  1    164 6.60
20  2    189 6.62
34  2    182 6.89
43  2    184 6.90
35  2    174 7.00
39  2    177 7.20
43  2    183 7.30
37  2    175 7.65
32  2    173 7.80
24  2    173 7.90
20  1    162 8.05
25  2    180 8.10
22  2    173 8.70
25  2    171 9.45
```

Proceed to enter these data in the above way, including labels as first line using the Notepad facility of Windows with either spaces or tabs as delimiters between numbers in a file having lungcap.txt as its name. An alternate mode is to use Excel for data entry and then save the file with Save As and specifying the file form as tab delimited. This latter will also produce a file with a .txt extension on the filename. It will be assumed here that you save the file using lungcap as the main part of the filename. The file is to be saved in the working folder that you use for R.

Now startup R, and use the following commands to read the data table into a data frame using Lung.capacity as the name of the data frame and see the first six lines.

```
>Lung.capacity <- read.table("lungcap.txt",header=T)
>head(Lung.capacity)
```

References

Dalgaard P (2002) Introductory statistics with R. Springer

Venables W, Smith D (2004) An introduction to R (revised and updated). Published by Network Theory Ltd., 15 Royal Park, Bristol, BS8 3

Appendix 3
R~Workshop II—Data Exploration with R

This workshop assumes the following:

- That you have R installed on your computer;
- That you are using a Windows® PC computer;
- That you have the lungcap.txt data file from Workshop I in the working folder;
- That you know how to enter R commands and use R as a calculator;
- That you can use the R help facilities;
- That you are acquainted with naming of objects in R;
- That you are acquainted with the nature of vectors and data frames in R.

We focus here on accessing the information in a data file as an **R** data frame, declaring categorical variables as **R** factors, annotating your **R** session, obtaining summary information for a data frame, and making some simple graphical plots to help understand the general characteristics of the information in a data frame.

R Startup Folder

You should always do your **R** work in a folder of your own, using a different folder for each analysis project. You can change the working folder (dir) from the File menu in R.

Annotating the R Session

We begin by noting that # character has a special purpose in **R**. When a # appears on a line, anything following on the same line is treated as annotation and ignored by **R**. Accordingly, you can annotate your **R** session for later reference by making a # the first thing that you enter on the line. Of course, the **R** prompt will be the very first thing that actually appears on the line. Examples in this workshop will be annotated in this manner.

Reading Data Table and Declaring Numeric Coded Categorical Factors

```
> # Read lungcap file into LungCap frame with column names.
> LungCap <- read.table("lungcap.txt",header=T)
> # Get list of variable names in LungCap data frame.
> names(LungCap)
[1] "age"    "sex"    "height" "tlc"
> # Declare sex as factor with 1 and 2 as level codes.
> LungCap$sex <- factor(LungCap$sex,levels=1:2)
> # Assign category labels to levels of sex.
> levels(LungCap$sex) <- c("F","M")
> #
```

Requesting a General Statistical Summary

A statistical summary for the variables in the data frame is requested as follows:

```
> # Request general statistical summary for data frame.
> summary(LungCap)
      age         sex       height           tlc
 Min.   :11.00   F:16   Min.   :138.0   Min.   :3.400
 1st Qu.:20.75   M:16   1st Qu.:159.5   1st Qu.:4.760
 Median :28.50          Median :170.0   Median :6.150
 Mean   :28.41          Mean   :167.4   Mean   :6.088
 3rd Qu.:35.00          3rd Qu.:175.5   3rd Qu.:7.225
 Max.   :52.00          Max.   :189.0   Max.   :9.450
```

For a regular numeric variable, you get the minimum, first quartile, median, mean, third quartile, and maximum. For a factor, you get a count of each level. Note that using the summary() command this way will print the results, but then they are gone. To save the results, we could have put them into an object—in which case we would need to enter the name of the object as if it were a command in order to get a printout.

```
> #
> LungCap.summary <- summary(LungCap)
> LungCap.summary
```

By using the attributes(LungCap.summary) command, we could determine that LungCap.summary belongs to a "table" class of **R** objects. Note that LungCap. summary is all one name, with the period only serving to improve readability. If we are going to do much work with a data frame, we should attach() the data frame to make its component variables accessible by variable name instead of the more cumbersome DataFrame$VariableName protocol. However, we should only have one data frame attached at a time. We should detach() the current one before attaching another one.

```
> # Attach the data frame for direct access to names.
> attach(LungCap)
```

Now, we can request particular statistics for a variable individually, for example:

```
> mean(age)
[1] 28.40625
> median(height)
[1] 170
```

The statistics reported by the summary() command are all measures of location (position) in the frequency distributions of the variables. To get standard deviations as a measure of variability, we could use the sd() command.

```
> sd(LungCap[-2])
      age      height         tlc
10.518369 11.948647    1.623537
```

Since the sex variable is a categorical factor, it must be omitted or there would be an error. There is a var() command for getting variances, but this is not convenient for present purposes since it produces a variance–covariance matrix instead of a variance vector. Since sd(LungCap[-2]) is a vector, we can get variances as the squares of the respective elements.

```
> sd(LungCap[-2])^2
       age       height          tlc
110.636089 142.770161     2.635871
```

Note that arithmetic and algebra are done element-by-element on vectors. So that the result would be more easily interpretable for later reference, it would have been better to put this computation into an object that we might call LungCap.variances and then display this object.

```
> #
> LungCap.variances <- sd(LungCap[-2])^2
> LungCap.variances
       age       height          tlc
110.636089 142.770161     2.635871
```

R has an internal spreadsheet editor if we want to examine the individual values of a data frame without cluttering up our output. We can put the output of the editor into an object called something like Temp and then remove the Temp object with the rm(Temp) command when we close the editor.

```
> Temp <- edit(LungCap)
> rm(Temp)
```

If we had actually wanted to change a value in LungCap with the editor, then the object containing the output of editor would not be disposable. If you intend to replace the original LungCap with the changed version, you can put the output back into LungCap again. To avoid lots of confusion, however, you should detach(LungCap) beforehand. You can then attach(LungCap) again after leaving the editor.

Reordering

We can create a version of LungCap that is ordered by age (column 1) and call it LungCapOrdr with the following command:

```
> LungCapOrdr <- LungCap[order(LungCap[,1]),1:4]
```

Although this appears somewhat messy, the form must be followed and the parts understood. Since we can order all or part of LungCap, the ordering is given as an indexed component of LungCap using square brackets. This component consists of an ordering of LungCap indexed on column 1 with square brackets again denoting an index. The ordered component of LungCap is to include columns 1 through 4, all of which are ordered according to the age values in column 1. An inverted ordering can be given as:

```
> LungCapInvOrdr <- LungCap[rev(order(LungCap[,1])),1:4]
```

Ordering is different from ranking, since ordering rearranges the values whereas ranking gives rank numbers. To illustrate this, let us create a small vector called Example and obtain its ranks.

```
> # Make a small vector called Example.
> Example <- c(4,2,8,6,9,5)
> Example
[1] 4 2 8 6 9 5
> # Find the rank numbers.
> rank(Example)
[1] 2 1 5 4 6 3
```

We can also use conditional relations in extracting components of a data frame. With the LungCap data frame being attached, let us get the cases with age greater than 40.

```
> # Get LungCap cases with age>40.
> LungCapOld <- LungCap[age>40,]
> LungCapOld
   age sex height  tlc
14  52   M     178 5.77
15  46   F     169 5.80
22  43   M     184 6.90
25  43   M     183 7.30
```

Generic Graphics

We next experiment with generic graphics for exploratory examination of data. Alternatives are available for displaying distribution of data. We illustrate with the age variable of the lung capacity data, and you can practice on the height and total lung capacity (tlc) variables. Remember that accessing variables directly by name requires that the data frame be attached

A histogram is a conventional way displaying distribution of data, and it is obtained with the hist() command.

```
> # Get a histogram of the age variable.
> hist(age)
```

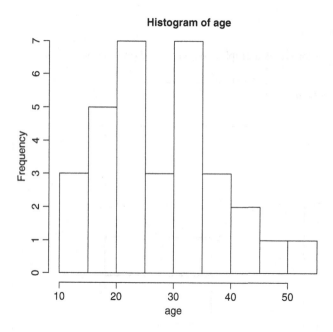

A second way is to make a stem-and-leaf diagram using the stem() command that shows the distributions of the first two digits (orders of magnitude) in the data.

```
> # Get a stem-and-leaf diagram of the age distribution.
> stem(age)
```

```
The decimal point is 1 digit(s) to the right of the |
1 | 124
1 | 666
2 | 0011234
2 | 5589
3 | 02234
3 | 55579
4 | 033
4 | 6
5 | 2
```

So, for example, there are three cases having 16 as the age.

```
> LungCap[age==16,]
  age sex height  tlc
4  16   F    156 3.90
6  16   F    157 4.10
8  16   M    152 4.55
```

A box plot provides a graphic display based on order statistics.

```
> #Get a box plot of the age data.
> boxplot(age)
```

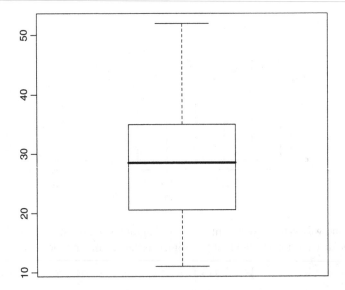

If no optional specifications are given to the boxplot function, the heavy horizontal line in the central box is the median, the bottom of the central box is the first quartile, the top of the central box is the third quartile, the "whiskers" extend to the most extreme value that is within 1.5 times the IQR inter-quartile range (third quartile–first quartile). More extreme values would be shown as outliers by plotting individual points.

Now, we obtain a qq-plot for judging the degree of normality.

```
> #Get a qq-plot for indicating degree of normality.
> qqnorm(age)
> #Add a qqline.
> qqline(age)
```

In this kind of plot, the plotted points for a normally distributed variable will fall on a straight line. Departures from a straight line indicate non-normal distribution. The qqline on the graph passes through the first and third quartiles.

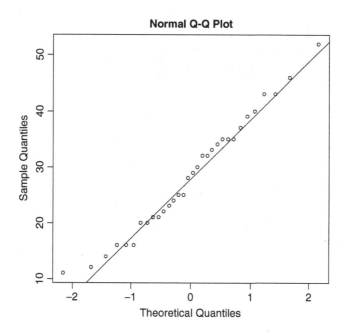

We finish with a scatterplot of height on *Y*-axis against age on the *X*-axis.

```
> #Scatterplot of height as Y against age as X.
> plot(age,height)
```

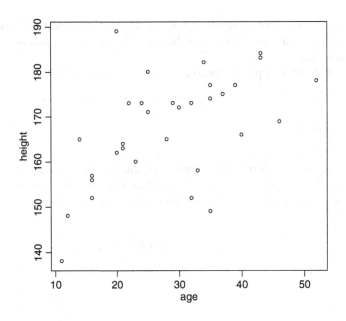

Appendix 4
R~Workshop III—Data Relations

This workshop assumes that you are acquainted with starting **R**, entering commands, reading data frames from files, and doing exploratory data summaries with **R**. In this workshop, we consider investigation of relationships between variables.

Illustrative Data

As in workshop II, we will use data on total lung capacity presented by Altman (1991) Practical statistics for medical research (Exercise 12.5, 10.1) published by Chapman & Hall that is recorded in a lungcap.txt file as per workshop II. Therefore, we begin by reading this into a data frame, checking the variable names, declaring a factor, requesting a summary, and then attaching the data frame.

```
> LungCap <- read.table("lungcap.txt",header=T)
> names(LungCap)
[1] "age"     "sex"     "height" "tlc"
> LungCap$sex <- factor(LungCap$sex,levels=1:2)
> levels(LungCap$sex) <- c("F","M")
> summary(LungCap)
      age          sex       height           tlc
 Min.   :11.00   F:16   Min.   :138.0   Min.   :3.400
 1st Qu.:20.75   M:16   1st Qu.:159.5   1st Qu.:4.760
 Median :28.50          Median :170.0   Median :6.150
 Mean   :28.41          Mean   :167.4   Mean   :6.088
 3rd Qu.:35.00          3rd Qu.:175.5   3rd Qu.:7.225
 Max.   :52.00          Max.   :189.0   Max.   :9.450
> attach(LungCap)
```

Correlation

For purposes of illustration, we focus first on the relationship between age and height. It always helps in this regard to have a visual perspective, so we first make a scatterplot of age on the horizontal (*X*) axis and height on the vertical (*Y*) axis.

```
> plot(age,height)
```

Note that the first argument for the plot command goes on the horizontal axis and the second goes on the vertical axis. By using optional additional arguments to the plot command, we could control and customize most of the aspects of the plot. The command in its simple form will not put a main title on the plot. We add an argument to put on a main title:

```
> plot(age,height,main="Joint Distribution of Ht and Age")
```

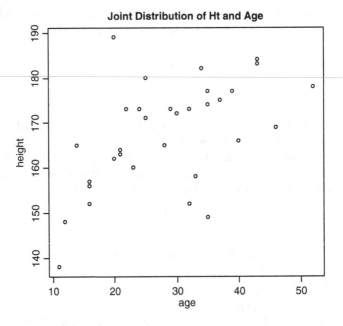

The usual quantitative measure of association is called correlation, and this can be computed with the cor() command in **R**.

```
> # Compute Pearson correlation coefficient.
> cor(age,height)
[1] 0.531639
```

Formally, the Pearson correlation coefficient is the covariance between standardized variables. A variable is standardized by rescaling each case by first subtracting the mean and then dividing by the standard deviation. Any standardized variable has mean of zero and variance of one. The (Pearson) correlation coefficient for a sample is usually denoted by **r** and is constrained to lie between negative one and positive one, inclusive. A correlation of zero indicates no apparent (linear) relationship; whereas a positive 1.0 indicates a perfect direct linear relationship, and a negative 1.0 indicates perfect inverse linear relationship. Moving away from zero, the scatter about a line becomes less.

A large-sample standard error of the bivariate correlation coefficient for testing the null hypothesis of **r**=0 can be computed as follows with $n-2$ degrees of freedom.

```
> AgeHtCor <- cor(age,height)
> Ncases <- length(age)
> Ncases
[1] 32
> CorStdErr <- sqrt((1.0 - AgeHtCor^2)/(Ncases - 2))
> CorStdErr
[1] 0.1546351
```

Dividing the correlation coefficient by its standard error gives a t-statistic having $n-2=30$ degrees of freedom. The two-tailed probability can be obtained by subtracting the cumulative probability of the t-distribution from 1.0 and then doubling it. The cumulative probability is given by the pt() function.

```
> tstat <- AgeHtCor/CorStdErr
> tstat
[1] 3.438024
> pt(tstat,30)
[1] 0.99913
> 2.0*(1.0 - pt(tstat,30))
[1] 0.001740163
```

This is highly significant, so there is strong evidence for an association between age and height. We would, of course, expect that people do not keep growing linearly much beyond 20 years of age—so there is good reason to anticipate a nonlinear relationship. For a nonlinear but nondecreasing relationship, we should use the Spearman rank correlation coefficient instead of the Pearson version. The Spearman version is obtained by converting the data to rank numbers, and then doing computation on the ranks instead of the raw data.

```
> # Compute the Spearman rank correlation coefficient.
> cor(age,height,method="spearman")
[1] 0.5574132
```

The fact that Spearman version is larger than the Pearson version supports nonlinearity.

The cor() function will compute correlations between the several variables in a data frame all at once to produce a correlation matrix. However, factors must be considered as effectively being missing data. A matrix is a row–column array of values, all of which are basically of the same type. A correlation matrix has the same number of rows and columns, and it is symmetric about the upper-left to lower-right diagonal—so it has redundant entries. The elements on the diagonal represent a relation of a variable with itself, which is always perfect so 1.0 appears on the entire diagonal. We delete the Not-Applicable factor entries to obtain the matrix for other variables.

```
> CorMatrx <- cor(LungCap,use="pairwise.complete.obs")
Warning message:
NAs introduced by coercion
> #
> CorMatrx
             age sex   height       tlc
age    1.0000000  NA 0.531639 0.2323495
sex          NA  NA       NA        NA
height 0.5316390  NA 1.000000 0.6957020
tlc    0.2323495  NA 0.695702 1.0000000
> # Delete NA factor elements in row 2 and column 2.
> CorMatrx <- CorMatrx[-2,-2]
> CorMatrx
             age   height       tlc
age    1.0000000 0.531639 0.2323495
height 0.5316390 1.000000 0.6957020
tlc    0.2323495 0.695702 1.0000000
```

Probability Distributions

This is a convenient place to note that several other probability distributions are available in **R** to be used in a manner like we used the t-distribution through the pt() function. The version of a function beginning with the letter p is used to find probabilities. The version of the function beginning with the letter q is used for the inverse purpose to find quantiles of the distribution corresponding to specified cumulative probabilities. Among these are:

normal using _norm()

lognormal using _lnorm()

t using _t()

F using _f()

chi-square using _chisq()

binomial using _binom()

Poisson using _pois()

uniform using _unif()

exponential using _exp()

gamma using _gamma()

beta using _beta()

Regression and Modeling of Relations

In regression and related analysis, we use one or more so-called independent variables to account for (model) the variation in a dependent variable. The independent variables are effectively the hypothesized drivers of the relationship, and the dependent variable is the response. **R** has elaborate facilities for specifying and producing such models, with the tilde ~ being used as a short-hand for "modeled by". The lm() or linear model facility is a primary one for such purposes.

Let us begin by modeling height as a simple linear function of age.

```
> HtAgeModl <- lm(height~age)
> HtAgeModl

Call:
lm(formula = height ~ age)

Coefficients:
(Intercept)          age
   150.2821       0.6039
```

HtAgeModl is now a "model object" in R that contains the fitted model as:

ht = 150.2821 + 0.6039age

along with ancillary information that can be extracted by summary(HtAgeModl) command. We now show this model line on a scatterplot.

```
> abline(HtAgeModl)
```

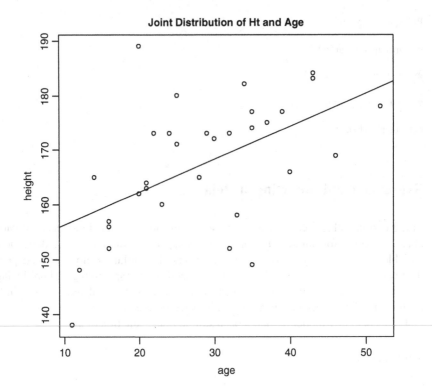

To predict height from a given age with our simple model, we find the age on the
X-axis, then move up vertically to the line, and across to the height on the Y-axis.
If we request a summary of our model, we get:

```
> summary(HtAgeModl)
Call:
lm(formula = height ~ age)

Residuals:
    Min     1Q  Median      3Q     Max
-22.420  -5.116   1.704   5.780  26.639

Coefficients:
             Estimate Std. Error t value Pr(>|t|)
(Intercept) 150.2821     5.3110  28.297  < 2e-16 ***
age           0.6039     0.1757   3.438  0.00174 **
---

Signif. codes:  0 '***' 0.001 '**' 0.01 '*' 0.05 '.' 0.1 '
 ' 1

Residual standard error: 10.29 on 30 degrees of freedom
Multiple R-Squared: 0.2826,     Adjusted R-squared: 0.2587
F-statistic: 11.82 on 1 and 30 DF,  p-value: 0.00174
```

We note that the "Multiple R-squared" of 0.2826 is the square of the value 0.5316 that we obtained earlier for the Pearson correlation coefficient with the cor() function. A residual is the difference between an actual value of height and its value as predicted from our age model, or the vertical distance from the point down to the trend line. A standard error is given for each coefficient, and dividing the coefficient by the standard error gives the t-value, both of which are highly significant in our case.

We can get a vector object of predictions for all the data cases with the command:

```
> HtAgePred <- predict(HtAgeModl)
```

And then, we obtain a vector object of case residuals as:

```
> HtAgeRes <- height - HtAgePred
```

We can then plot actual values against predictions:

```
> plot(HtAgePred,height)
```

The fitted() command is an alternative to predict() with regard to observed cases.

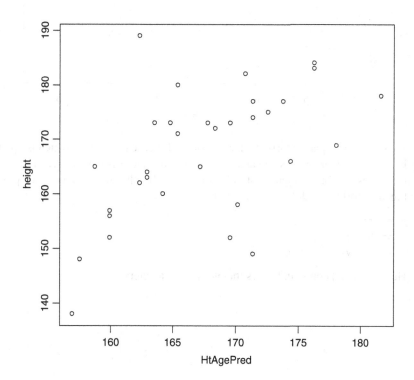

We can also plot residuals against case numbers (index), where we note that omitting the second argument to the plot() command will give a plot on the *Y*-axis versus case index number on the *X*-axis.

```
> plot(HtAgeRes)
```

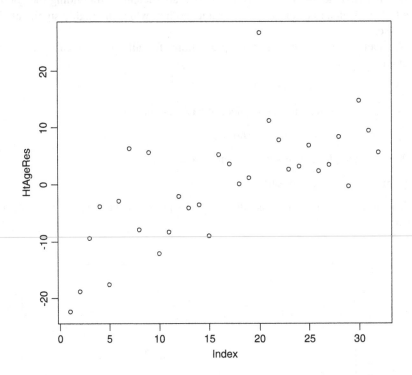

We should note particularly the large residual for case number 20 which is up all by itself. The modern regression analyst would also want a display of special regression diagnostics for residuals that is best obtained by altering the layout for plots and then restoring the default afterwards.

```
> par(mfrow=c(2,2),mex=0.6)
> plot(HtAgeMod1)
> par(mfrow=c(1,1),mex=1)
```

Here, the par() command alters the plotting parameters.

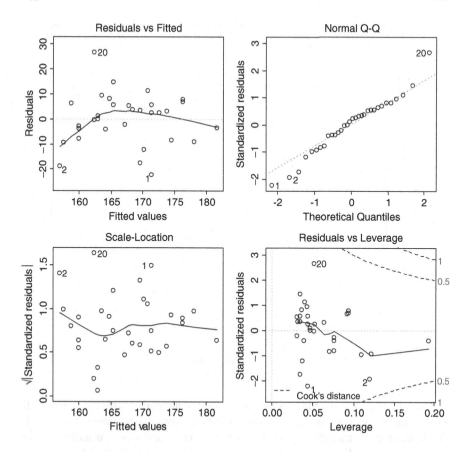

We should not be satisfied with a model that is under suspicion for potential improvement, as we suspect from cessation of height growth with advancing age—particularly, when the diagnostic plots indicate problems with outliers.

Let us return to the plot of actual against predicted heights, and sketch in an empirical trend with the lowess() command (missing data not allowed). We also take advantage of the identify() capability in the plotting facility to check on points which we find of interest. When this is invoked, pressing the left mouse button on a point in the plot will label it. When all points of interest have been labeled, then press the right mouse button to stop.

```
> plot(HtAgePred,height)
> lines(lowess(HtAgePred,height))
> identify(HtAgePred,height)
[1]   1   5  20
```

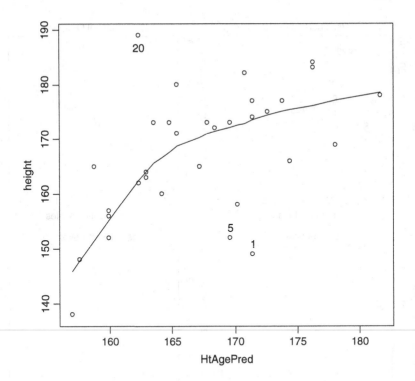

This plot shows both evidence of outliers and nonlinearity, with cases 1 and 20 also being flagged as outliers by the foregoing regression diagnostics panel. Therefore, further modeling work is needed. A next step would usually involve dropping some outliers and using a quadratic polynomial predictor. A model for quadratic polynomial could be:

```
> QuadModl <- lm(height~ age + I(age^2))
```

The I() designation is used as a wrapper to keep what is inside from being interpreted as modeling symbols instead of squaring age. It is possible to experiment with many models very quickly in **R** by using the following modeling symbology:

```
+ means include a term in the model;
- means delete a term from the model;
* means include interaction terms;
/ means nesting of terms in the model;
| means conditioning of terms in the model;
: means interaction.
```

Appendix 5
R~Workshop IV—Analysis of Variance and Covariance

This workshop assumes that you are acquainted with starting **R**, entering commands, reading data frames from files, doing exploratory data summaries with **R**, and fitting basic regression models with the lm() facility of **R**. In this workshop, we look at analysis of variance (AOV or ANOVA) models using categorical factors and analysis of covariance (ANCOVA) models that combine categorical factors and regression variables.

Single-Factor Models

A single-factor model looks for differences in a response variable associated with levels of a categorical factor variable. We can have different numbers of cases for the different levels in this relatively simple case. However, lack of such balance among levels will considerably complicate multifactor situations. We start again with the data on total lung capacity presented by Altman (1991). Practical statistics for medical research (Exercise 12.5, 10.1) published by Chapman & Hall as recorded in lungcap.txt file from preceding workshops. Thus, we initially read into a data frame, check variable names, declare sex factor, request a summary, and attach the frame.

```
> LungCap <- read.table("lungcap.txt",header=T)
> names(LungCap)
[1] "age"     "sex"     "height" "tlc"
> Check <- edit(LungCap)
> rm(Check)
> LungCap$sex <- factor(LungCap$sex,levels=1:2)
> levels(LungCap$sex) <- c("Female","Male")
> summary(LungCap)
      age             sex         height           tlc
 Min.   :11.00   Female:16   Min.   :138.0   Min.   :3.400
 1st Qu.:20.75   Male  :16   1st Qu.:159.5   1st Qu.:4.760
 Median :28.50               Median :170.0   Median :6.150
 Mean   :28.41               Mean   :167.4   Mean   :6.088
 3rd Qu.:35.00               3rd Qu.:175.5   3rd Qu.:7.225
 Max.   :52.00               Max.   :189.0   Max.   :9.450
> attach(LungCap)
```

The editing of LungCap into the Check object was done to see what levels occur in the sex variable so that the factor declaration can be accomplished. The Check object is then removed with the rm() command.

We proceed to do the simplest kind of AOV with a single factor having two levels, which could also be approached with a two-sample t-test. The F-statistic from AOV will be the same as the square of the t-statistic in a two-sample test. Let us do the two-sample t-test as a preliminary, and also plot parallel box plots. The response variable is total lung capacity (tlc) and the factor is sex.

```
> TwoSample <- t.test(tlc~sex)
> TwoSample

        Welch Two Sample t-test

data:  tlc by sex
t = -3.6693, df = 29.703, p-value = 0.0009493
alternative hypothesis: true difference in means is not
equal to 0
95 percent confidence interval:
 -2.7691965 -0.7883035
sample estimates:
mean in group Female    mean in group Male
            5.198125              6.976875
```

The difference is very highly significant with females having lower tlc than males.

```
> boxplot(tlc~sex)
```

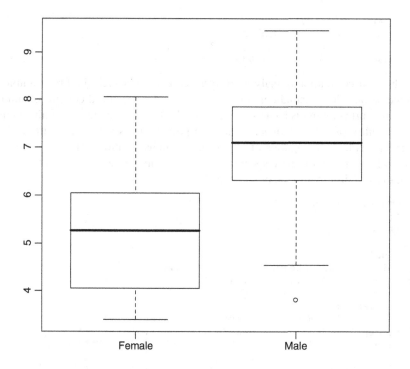

Notice that the male having lung capacity of 3.8 is considered an outlier, whereas this is not an outlier value for females.

```
> OneWayAOV <- aov(tlc~sex)
> OneWayAOV
Call:
   aov(formula = tlc ~ sex)

Terms:
                        sex Residuals
Sum of Squares     25.31161   56.40039
Deg. of Freedom           1         30

Residual standard error: 1.371136
Estimated effects may be unbalanced
```

The immediate result of the aov() facility is information on sum of squares and degrees of freedom without even a test statistic. An F-statistic can be obtained by dividing each sum of squares by its degrees of freedom to get the respective mean squares, and then dividing the mean square for sex by the mean square for residuals to give F=13. 4635 which is the square of the earlier t-statistic apart from rounding. However, the usual summary() command will give us a more complete analysis of variance table.

```
> summary(OneWayAOV)
          Df Sum Sq Mean Sq F value     Pr(>F)
sex        1 25.312  25.312  13.464 0.0009392 ***
Residuals 30 56.400   1.880
```

This is a conventional analysis of variance table in which the first column is source of variation, second column is degrees of freedom, third column is sum of squares, fourth column is mean square, fifth column is F-statistic, and sixth column is probability of the F-statistic. Again, the probability is same as for the earlier t-statistic aside from vagaries of computational considerations. However, there is still no information on the respective response means by level. To get at this, we need to use a different mode of summary.

```
> summary.lm(OneWayAOV)
Call:
aov(formula = tlc ~ sex)

Residuals:
    Min      1Q  Median      3Q     Max
-3.1769 -1.0072  0.1231  0.8481  2.8519

Coefficients:
            Estimate Std. Error t value Pr(>|t|)
(Intercept)   5.1981     0.3428  15.164 1.31e-15 ***
sexMale       1.7788     0.4848   3.669  0.00094 ***
---
Signif. codes: 0 '***' 0.001 '**' 0.01 '*' 0.05 '.' 0.1 ' '

Residual standard error: 1.371 on 30 degrees of freedom
Multiple R-Squared: 0.3098,     Adjusted R-squared: 0.2868
F-statistic: 13.46 on 1 and 30 DF,  p-value: 0.0009392
```

Still it is not clear, however, what the means of the response variable are for the respective levels of sex. A clue will make this clear. Notice that the Intercept is the same as the mean for Female given by the earlier two-sample test. The sexMale coefficient is the difference between the mean for Males and the mean for Females. Thus,

```
Male mean = 5.1981 + 1.7788 = 6.9769
```

The fact that the sexMale coefficient is positive indicates that it must be added to the Intercept mean. The level chosen to serve as the Intercept is the one for which the name is alphabetically first—in this case Female. Note also that standard error given for sexMale is the standard error of a difference, not of the sexMale mean itself.

Two-Way Factorial AOV

For convenience of illustration, we now switch to a fictitious dataset created to show features of a two-way factorial arrangement. There are two factors, which we will call simply FactrA and FactrB. FactrA has three levels, which we will call A1, A2, and A3. FactrB has two levels, which we will call B1 and B2. The response variable

will be called OutCome. A listing of data to be entered in a file named whatif.txt is
as follows.

```
  Afactr Bfactr OutCome
1    1      1     35
2    1      1     30
3    1      1     27
4    1      2     22
5    1      2     23
6    1      2     24
7    2      1     71
8    2      1     69
9    2      1     75
10   2      2     52
11   2      2     46
12   2      2     68
13   3      1     98
14   3      1     96
15   3      1     90
16   3      2     76
17   3      2     71
18   3      2     73
```

The **R** commands to bring this in as a data frame called WhatIf are as follows:

```
> WhatIf <- read.table("whatif.txt",header=T)
> names(WhatIf)
[1] "Afactr"  "Bfactr"  "OutCome"
> WhatIf$Afactr <- factor(WhatIf$Afactr,levels=1:3)
> WhatIf$Bfactr <- factor(WhatIf$Bfactr,levels=1:2)
> levels(WhatIf$Afactr) <- c("A1","A2","A3")
> levels(WhatIf$Bfactr) <- c("B1","B2")
> summary(WhatIf)
Afactr Bfactr     OutCome
 A1:6   B1:9   Min.    :22.00
 A2:6   B2:9   1st Qu.:31.25
 A3:6          Median :68.50
               Mean    :58.11
               3rd Qu.:74.50
               Max.    :98.00
> attach(WhatIf)
```

Instead of going through the mechanics of extracting the means for treatments
from model output, let us use the tapply() command to create a table of means
before doing the analysis of variance.

```
> tapply(OutCome,list(Afactr,Bfactr),mean)
         B1         B2
A1 30.66667  23.00000
A2 71.66667  55.33333
A3 94.66667  73.33333
```

There are three replications for each of the treatment combinations, so this is a
"balanced" design that is relatively straightforward to analyze. There are three types
of "effects" to be investigated: an overall (or main) effect of FactrA, an overall

(or main) effect of FactrB, and "interaction" effects of FactrA and FactrB. The interaction is concerned with whether the effect of FactrA may be specific to the level of FactrB and vice versa. The degrees of freedom for the FactrA main effect is one less than the levels $(3-1=2)$, and for the FactrB main effect $(2-1=1)$. The degrees of freedom for interaction is $(\text{Alevels}-1)\times(\text{Blevels}-1)=(3-1)\times(2-1)=2$. The remainder of the $n-1=18-1=17$ total degrees of freedom are called "error" degrees of freedom because they reflect variation among the experimental units that are not within the capability of the investigator to control without better facilities and more uniform units.

We proceed to compute a "maximal model" including all of the potential effects.

```
> MaxFactrModl <- aov(OutCome~Afactr*Bfactr)
> summary(MaxFactrModl)
              Df  Sum Sq Mean Sq  F value      Pr(>F)
Afactr         2 10065.4  5032.7 168.0686 1.677e-09 ***
Bfactr         1  1027.6  1027.6  34.3154 7.742e-05 ***
Afactr:Bfactr  2   143.4    71.7   2.3952    0.1333
Residuals     12   359.3    29.9
```

We see that each of our "effects" has a line in the AOV table and the "Residuals" comprise entirely of the "error" degrees of freedom. Both of the "main" effects are very highly significant, but the probability of observing this kind of interaction by chance is more than double the usual 5% criterion. Since we should not recognize effects that are not significant in our model, it is appropriate to formulate a "reduced" model without the interaction which will incorporate the degrees of freedom for interaction into residuals.

```
> ReduFactrModl <- aov(OutCome~ Afactr + Bfactr)
> summary(ReduFactrModl)
            Df  Sum Sq Mean Sq F value      Pr(>F)
Afactr       2 10065.4  5032.7 140.138 5.516e-10 ***
Bfactr       1  1027.6  1027.6  28.613 0.0001026 ***
Residuals   14   502.8    35.9
```

We now have an appropriate model in which all of the recognized effects are significant. Note the difference in the way the two models are specified. The * in the first model says to recognize both main effects and interaction. The + sign in the second model adds only the Bfactr main effect to the Afactr main effect.

As a matter of curiosity, let us change the OutCome values where Afactr="A1" and Bfactr="B1" from 35 30 27 to 10 15 12 and then do a new maximal model.

```
> NewModl <- aov(OutCome~ Afactr*Bfactr)
> summary(NewModl)
              Df  Sum Sq Mean Sq F value      Pr(>F)
Afactr         2 13842.1  6921.1 244.753 1.877e-10 ***
Bfactr         1   364.5   364.5  12.890 0.0037117 **
Afactr:Bfactr  2   889.0   444.5  15.719 0.0004445 ***
Residuals     12   339.3    28.3
```

Now all three types of effects are significant, with the significant interaction indicating that Afactr and Bfactr behave differently in combination than separately.

```
> tapply(OutCome,list(Afactr,Bfactr),mean)
        B1        B2
A1 12.33333 23.00000
A2 71.66667 55.33333
A3 94.66667 73.33333
```

The mean of B1 is now less than B2 when in company with A1, but otherwise the mean of B1 is greater than that of B2.

Split-Plot, Nesting, and Random Effects

What is all too often not appreciated is that the perspective on data and nature of modeling confers the meaning, rather than necessarily the numbers themselves. This is well illustrated by the difference between factorial structure and split-plot structure for data. In a factorial structure, the experimental units are randomized individually so that all have the same chance of receiving every treatment combination.

In a split-plot approach, the different treatment factors are randomized in stages and differ in the scope of units at each stage. For example, we might have larger plots for Afactr than for Bfactr, with Bfactr levels being allocated to plots that are half the size for Afactr levels. Thus, Afactr is randomly allocated to large plots, and then a random choice is made as to which half of the Afactr plot gets which level of Bfactr. Note carefully, however, that each large Afactr plot still gets the same two Bfactr levels. This calls for a column in the data file to identify a replicate and inclusion of an Error() specification in the model, since different effects have different residual mean square denominators for the F-tests. A nested design might differ from a split-plot in that measurements are taken on subplots of large plots without having exactly the same set of subplot conditions in each larger plot. This would entail random effects at the subplot level and a mixed-effects model. This underscores the importance of conceiving the model in advance and learning appropriately sophisticated modeling features of R.

Analysis of Covariance

An analysis of covariance (ANCOVA) model is one which has both categorical factors and regular measured variables that are (suspected of being) related to the response variable. For a basic encounter with this type of model, we refer again to the total lung capacity data with which we began this workshop. The variables are age, sex, height, and total lung capacity (tlc). We might be interested again in knowing whether there is a difference for sex beyond any differences associated with heights. This is a dual problem in regression and analysis of variance, since we consider the possibility that each sex may have a different regression line for tlc on height; that is, differing in either slope or intercept. This illustrates in more detail the protocol of starting with a maximal model and removing effects that are not significant in reduced models. We will not make any use of the age variable for present purposes. We approach this more like a regression analysis, since we will use the lm() linear model facility instead of the aov() facility in **R**. Accordingly, we begin with a maximal model that allows for difference in both slope and intercept by sex—that is, interaction of sex and height with regard to tlc.

```
> LungCap <- read.table("lungcap.txt",header=T)
> names(LungCap)
[1] "age"     "sex"      "height" "tlc"
> LungCap$sex <- factor(LungCap$sex,levels=1:2)
> levels(LungCap$sex) <- c("Female","Male")
> attach(LungCap)
> MaxModl <- lm(tlc~height*sex)
> summary.aov(MaxModl)
             Df Sum Sq Mean Sq F value    Pr(>F)
height        1 39.549  39.549 28.4717 1.108e-05 ***
sex           1  3.245   3.245  2.3363    0.1376
height:sex    1  0.025   0.025  0.0176    0.8953
Residuals    28 38.894   1.389
```

This leads us to believe that height is a significant consideration in relation to total lung capacity, but that sex is not. This is interesting since we earlier saw that sex was significant without considering height. The other way we could have specified the model is with sex before height

```
> MxModl <- lm(tlc~sex*height)
> summary.aov(MxModl)
             Df Sum Sq Mean Sq F value    Pr(>F)
sex           1 25.312  25.312 18.2222 0.0002036 ***
height        1 17.482  17.482 12.5858 0.0013924 **
sex:height    1  0.025   0.025  0.0176 0.8952822
Residuals    28 38.894   1.389
```

This reverse order casts a different light on the matter, since sex and height both appear to be significant. The moral of the story here is that order of consideration makes a difference in analysis of covariance, and this is also true for analysis of variance when balance is lacking. However, we still need to decide what to do about it. A preliminary step is to eliminate the interaction that is not significant in either model, and which corresponds to differences in slopes of the regression of tlc on height.

```
> ReducModlA <- lm(tlc~ height + sex)
> summary.aov(ReducModlA)
             Df Sum Sq Mean Sq F value    Pr(>F)
height        1 39.549  39.549 29.4699 7.711e-06 ***
sex           1  3.245   3.245  2.4182    0.1308
Residuals    29 38.918   1.342
```

```
> ReducModlB <- lm(tlc~ sex + height)
> summary.aov(ReducModlB)
             Df Sum Sq Mean Sq F value    Pr(>F)
sex           1 25.312  25.312 18.861 0.0001566 ***
height        1 17.482  17.482 13.027 0.0011423 **
Residuals    29 38.918   1.342
```

   With the reduced model in either order, it seems clear that height is significant. Sex is not significant when considered after height, but it is before. The logical conclusion is the effect of sex is expressed as difference in height, and height makes a difference with respect to lung capacity. In other words, the linkage of sex to lung capacity is through height. We can do one more thing, which is to fit a further reduced model with height alone.

```
> ReducMod1C <- lm(tlc~height)
> summary.aov(ReducMod1C)
           Df Sum Sq Mean Sq F value      Pr(>F)
height      1 39.549  39.549  28.140 9.853e-06 ***
Residuals  30 42.163   1.405
```

   We note that the aov version of summary does not give us the coefficients of the regression line, so we request a simple summary.

```
> summary(ReducMod1C)
Call:
lm(formula = tlc ~ height)

Residuals:
    Min     1Q  Median      3Q     Max
-2.1614 -0.6594 -0.2387  0.8281  3.0257

Coefficients:
             Estimate Std. Error t value Pr(>|t|)
(Intercept) -9.74025    2.99108  -3.256   0.0028 **
height       0.09453    0.01782   5.305 9.85e-06 ***

Residual standard error: 1.186 on 30 degrees of freedom
Multiple R-Squared: 0.484,       Adjusted R-squared: 0.4668
F-statistic: 28.14 on 1 and 30 DF,  p-value: 9.853e-06
```

   In more complex circumstances, the way to assess the effect of a model reduction is to compare the difference in residuals of the reduced and unreduced models by anova().

```
> anova(ReducMod1A,ReducMod1C)
Analysis of Variance Table

Model 1: tlc ~ height + sex
Model 2: tlc ~ height
  Res.Df    RSS Df Sum of Sq      F Pr(>F)
1     29 38.918
2     30 42.163 -1    -3.245 2.4182 0.1308
```

   The F-test for reduction indicates that the deleted component can be eliminated.

Appendix 6
Glossary of Names Designating Data (R Objects)

A – (In Chap. 14): Matrix for eigen extraction in discriminant (canonical axis) analysis.

B – (In Chap. 14): Between-groups (I, II, and III) covariance matrix.

B6C – Covariance matrix of BAMBI6 data frame.

B6E – **R** object containing eigen analysis for B6C matrix.

B6T – Matrix of eigenvectors for B6C matrix.

B6V – Vector of eigenvalues for B6C matrix.

B6Y – Data matrix of decorrelated (principal component score) data from transformation of BAMBI6 data.

BAMBI – Data frame containing bird and mammal biodiversity information for hexagonal cells in Pennsylvania, including hexagon identification numbers.

BAMBI6 – Data frame containing bird and mammal biodiversity information for hexagonal cells in Pennsylvania, but excluding hexagon identification numbers (same data as for BAMBIV data frame).

BAMBIR – Rank conversion of variates in BAMBIV data frame, with ranking being worst first.

BAMBIS – Standardized version of BAMBIV, whereby all variates have mean = 0 and standard deviation = 1.

BAMBISmean – Vector of mean values for standardized variates in BAMBIS data frame, used to show that all means are zero.

BAMBISpc – Data frame of principal component scores computed from BAMBIS data frame, with sign reversals for selected components.

BAMBISpca – Results of principal component analysis for BAMBIS data frame.

BAMBISsd – Vector of standard deviation values for standardized variates in BAMBIS data frame, used to show that all standard deviations are one.

BAMBIV – Data frame containing bird and mammal biodiversity information for hexagonal cells in Pennsylvania, but excluding hexagon identification numbers.

BAMBIVcv – Vector of coefficient of variation values of variates in BAMBIV data frame.

BAMBIVmean – Vector of mean values of variates in BAMBIV data frame.

BAMBIVsd – Vector of standard deviation values of variates in BAMBIV data frame.

Border – Data frame of border zone(s) for select sector in the Ridge & Valley Physiographic Region.

BorderIDs – Hexagon IDs for border zone(s) of select sector in the Ridge & Valley Physiographic Region.

BordrID – Hexagon IDs for border zone(s) of select sector regarding vertebrate species diversity in the Ridge & Valley Physiographic Region.

BorderOrd – Salient scaling for hexagons in border zone(s) of select sector in the Ridge & Valley Physiographic Region.

BordrOrd – Salient scaling for hexagons in border zones(s) of select sector regarding vertebrate species diversity in the Ridge & Valley Physiographic Region.

BorderRnks – Place rankings for indicators in border zone(s) of select sector in the Ridge & Valley Physiographic Region.

BordrRnks – Place rankings for indicators in border zone(s) of select sector regarding vertebrate species diversity in the Ridge & Valley Physiographic Region.

Bordrsp – Data frame of border zone(s) for select sector regarding vertebrate species diversity in the Ridge & Valley Physiographic Region.

BSE – **R** object containing eigen analysis for BSC matrix.

BSC – Covariance matrix of BAMBIS data frame, with BAMBIS data frame consisting of standardized data for BAMBI data frame. Therefore, BSC is also the correlation matrix for both BAMBI and BAMBIS data frames.

BST – Matrix of eigenvectors for BSC matrix.

BSV – Vector of eigenvalues for BSC matrix.

BSY – Data matrix of decorrelated (principal component score) data from transformation of BAMBIS data.

C – (In Chap. 14): Collective covariance matrix for BAMBIS data.

CasPlacRnk5 – Place rankings for cases on first five BAMBI variates with hexagon IDs.

CasRnkStat5 – Representative rank order statistics for cases on first five BAMBI variates with hexagon IDs.

Centr11 – Centroids (mean vectors) of 11 kmeans clusters of hexagons obtained from five principal components and expressed in terms of original measurement scales for variates.

Centr11PC – Centroids (mean vectors) of 11 kmeans clusters of hexagons obtained from five principal components and expressed in terms of (reoriented) principal component scores.

Centr11R – Centroids (mean vectors) of 11 kmeans clusters of hexagons obtained from principal components and expressed in terms of (worst first) ranks of variates.

Centr11S – Centroids (mean vectors) of 11 kmeans clusters of hexagons obtained from five principal components and expressed in terms of standardized measurement scales for variates.

Centr12 – Centroids (mean vectors) of 12 hierarchical clusters of hexagons obtained from five principal components and expressed in terms of original measurement scales for variates.

Centr12PC – Centroids (mean vectors) of 12 hierarchical clusters of hexagons obtained from five principal components and expressed in terms of (reoriented) principal component scores.

Centr12S – Centroids (mean vectors) of 12 hierarchical clusters of hexagons obtained from five principal components and expressed in terms of standardized measurement scales for variates.

ClusPC4 – Hierarchical clusters of hexagon cases based on four principal components.

ClusPC5 – Hierarchical clusters of hexagon cases based on five principal components.

ClusPC5hts – Top-down vector of disparities (dendrogram heights) between hierarchical clusters of hexagon cases based on five principal components.

ClusPC6 – Hierarchical clusters of hexagon cases based on six principal components.

CmplmntOrd – Salient scaling for hexagons regarding complementary vertebrate species diversity in the Ridge & Valley Physiographic Region.

Cntngn4 – Case place-rank data on first five variates of hexagons in contingent 4.

Cntngn4RR – Representative rank order statistics on first five variates for hexagons in contingent 4.

Cntngn5RR – Representative rank order statistics on first five variates for hexagons in contingent 5.

Cntngn6RR – Representative rank order statistics on first five variates for hexagons in contingent 6.

Cntngn7RR – Representative rank order statistics on first five variates for hexagons in contingent 7.

Cntngn10RR – Representative rank order statistics on first five variates for hexagons in contingent 10.

Cntngn5 – Case place-rank data on first five variates of hexagons in contingent 5.

Cntngn6 – Case place-rank data on first five variates of hexagons in contingent 6.

Cntngn7 – Case place-rank data on first five variates of hexagons in contingent 7.

Cntngn10 – Case place-rank data on first five variates of hexagons in contingent 10.

Cntngnt – Hexagon membership in 11 kmeans clusters based on five principal components and designated as factor levels for construction of classification tree.

CntngORD2 – ORDIT ordering of ORDIT orderings obtained from CntngOrdr2 data frame.

CntngOrdr2 – Data frame combining ORDIT ordering of contingents from quartiles of representative ranks with ORDIT orderings from three first PCO axes and three second PCO axes.

CntngnTree – Classification tree for 11 kmeans clusters (based on five principal components) in terms of hexagon variates on original measurement scales.

CONTINGN – Data frame of hexagon ID numbers and contingent numbers.

Contngt – Data frame of hexagon ID numbers and contingent numbers.

Dispar4pc – Euclidean distances between hexagon cases using four principal components.

Dispar5pc – Euclidean distances between hexagon cases using five principal components.

Dispar6pc – Euclidean distances between hexagon cases using six principal components.

Dist11 – Distances between centroids of 11 contingents of hexagons as scaled on original measurements.

Dist11R – Distances between centroids of 11 contingents of hexagons as scaled on place ranks.

Dist11S – Distances between centroids of 11 contingents of hexagons as scaled on standardized variates.

DistlData5 – Distal data for place ranks of first five variates of BAMBI data.

EcoLogic – Data frame of place ranks for ecological value and ecological sensitivity in Italian case study.

EcoSntvR – Place ranks of ecological sensitivity indicators for Italian case study.

EcoValuR – Place ranks of ecological value indicators for Italian cases study.

Egns – Eigen analysis for canonical (discriminant) axis analysis of Groups I, II, and III.

Hclus7 – Cluster membership of hexagons in seven hierarchical clusters obtained from five principal components.

H – (In Chap. 14): Transformation matrix for canonical (discriminant) variates of Groups I, II, and III.

Hclus12 – Cluster membership of hexagons in 12 hierarchical clusters obtained from five principal components.

HexNmbrs – Vector of hexagon ID numbers.

HexSet – Set of hexagons in select sector of Ridge & Valley Physiographic Region.

HexSetsp – Set of hexagons in select sector for vertebrate species richness and forest cover in Ridge & Valley Physiographic Region.

HumPresR – Place ranks of human pressure indicators for Italian case study.

ID4 – Hexagon ID numbers of hexagons in contingent 4.

ID5 – Hexagon ID numbers of hexagons in contingent 5.

ID6 – Hexagon ID numbers of hexagons in contingent 6.

ID7 – Hexagon ID numbers of hexagons in contingent 7.

ID10 – Hexagon ID numbers of hexagons in contingent 10.

IDTopRR – Hexagon ID numbers of hexagons in TopRR pool.

IDtops – Hexagon ID numbers of hexagons in Toppings pool.

IhexG – Canonical variates (discriminant axis) data for Group I.

IIhexG – Canonical variates (discriminant axis) data for Group II.

IIIhexG – Canonical variates (discriminant axis) data for Group III.

IhexS – Standardized data for hexagons in contingents 1, 2, and 3 as Group I.

IIhexS – Standardized data for hexagons in contingents 6, 8, 9, and 11 as Group II.

IIIhexS – Standardized data for hexagons in contingents 4, 5, 7, and 10 as Group III.

KdataPC5 – Principal component scores for first five (reoriented) components from BAMBISpc data frame.

KeyRnks11 – Representative ranks for 11 contingents across cases in contingent.

Klus11 – Hexagon membership in 11 kmeans clusters based on five principal components.

Klus11siz – Sizes of 11 kmeans clusters of hexagons based on five principal components.

Klus12 – Hexagon membership in 12 kmeans clusters based on five principal components.

Klus12siz – Sizes of 12 kmeans clusters of hexagons based on five principal components.

Kmeans11PC – Eleven kmeans clusters of hexagon cases based on five principal components, starting from centroids for 11 hierarchical clusters.

Kmeans12PC – Twelve kmeans clusters of hexagon cases based on five principal components, starting from centroids for 12 hierarchical clusters.

KstartPC5 – Centroids (mean vectors) of 12 hierarchical clusters of hexagons obtained from five principal components and expressed in terms of first five (reoriented) principal component scores.

KstrtPC5 – Centroids (mean vectors) of 11 hierarchical clusters (excluding hierarchical cluster 4 of KstartPC5).

L – (In Chap. 14): First for vector length, then for Cholesky decomposition of pooled within-groups (I, II, and III) covariance matrix.

M – (In Chap. 14): Diagonal matrix of multipliers for rescaling.

MisMatch – Median mismatches for place ranks of first five variates of BAMBI data.

MixModeRnks – Place ranks for centroids of 11 contingents on all six original BAMBI variates.

MixModeRnkS – Place ranks for centroids of 11 contingents on all six standardized BAMBI variates.

Nabors – K nearest neighbors for centroids of 11 contingents of hexagons using standardized measurement scales for the 6 variates.

NaborS – K nearest neighbors in principal coordinate space for centroids of 11 contingents of hexagons, with principal coordinates based on standardized variates.

NetFram – Network of neighbors on principal coordinates based on original scales of variates for centroids of contingents comprising PCOss subset.

NetFramS – Network of neighbors on principal coordinates based on standardized scales of variates for centroids of contingents comprising PCOss subset.

NetFrame – Network of neighbors on principal coordinates for centroids of 11 contingents of hexagons, with the principal coordinates based on original measurements.

NetFrameS – Network of neighbors on principal coordinates for centroids of 11 contingents of hexagons, with the principal coordinates based on standardized variates.

PCO11 – Principal coordinates for centroids of 11 contingents of hexagons by multidimensional scaling on original measurements.

PCO11R – Principal coordinates for centroids of 11 contingents of hexagons by multidimensional scaling on place-ranked variates.

PCO11S – Principal coordinates for centroids of 11 contingents of hexagons by multidimensional scaling on standardized measurements.

PCOblock – Rearrangement of PCOcombo to approximate block diagonal structure in for correlation matrix.

PCOcntr11 – Reoriented principal coordinates for centroids of 11 contingents of hexagons by multidimensional scaling on original measurements.

PCOcntr11R – Reoriented principal coordinates for centroids of 11 contingents of hexagons by multidimensional scaling on place-ranked variates.

PCOcntr11S – Reoriented principal coordinates for centroids of 11 contingents of hexagons by multidimensional scaling on standardized variates.

PCOcntr11ss – Centroids for skeletal subset for principal coordinates based on original variates.

PCOcntr11Sss – Centroids for skeletal subset for principal coordinates based on standardized variates.

PCOcombo – Data frame combining three sets of PCO variates.

PCOord1 – ORDIT ordering of contingents on three PCO axis 1 scales.

PCOord2 – ORDIT ordering of contingents on three PCO axis 2 scales.

ProdOrd4 – Salient scaling on first five variates for hexagons in contingent 4.

ProdOrd5 – Salient scaling on first five variates for hexagons in contingent 5.

ProdOrd6 – Salient scaling on first five variates for hexagons in contingent6.

ProdOrd7 – Salient scaling on first five variates for hexagons in contingent 7.

ProdOrd10 – Salient scaling on first five variates for hexagons in contingent 10.

ProdOrdTops – Salient scaling on first five variates for hexagons in Toppings pool.

PrOr4MnMdMx – Salient scaling on minimum, median, and maximum representative ranks for hexagons in contingent 4.

PrOr5MnMdMx – Salient scaling on minimum, median, and maximum representative ranks for hexagons in contingent 5.

PrOr6MnMdMx – Salient scaling on minimum, median, and maximum representative ranks for hexagons in contingent 6.

PrOr7MnMdMx – Salient scaling on minimum, median, and maximum representative ranks for hexagons in contingent 7.

PrOr10MnMdMx – Salient scaling on minimum, median and maximum representative ranks for hexagons in contingent 10.

PrOr4MnMx – Salient scaling on minimum rank and maximum rank for hexagons in contingent 4.

PrOr5MnMx – Salient scaling on minimum rank and maximum rank for hexagons in contingent 5.

PrOr6MnMx – Salient scaling on minimum rank and maximum rank for hexagons in contingent 6.

PrOr7MnMx – Salient scaling on minimum rank and maximum rank for hexagons in contingent 7.

PrOr10MnMx – Salient scaling on minimum rank and maximum rank for hexagons in contingent 10.

PrOrTopRRMnMx – Salient scaling on minimum and maximum representative ranks of first five variates for hexagons in TopRR pool.

PrOrTopRRMnMdMx – Salient scaling on minimum, median, and maximum representative ranks of first five variates for hexagons in TopRR pool.

Q – (In Chap. 14): Inverse of Cholesky decomposition of pooled within-groups (I, II, and III) covariance matrix.

Ranges – Vector of ranges for variates in BAMBIV data frame.

RVcmplmnt – Complementary ratings of hexagons in the Ridge & Valley Physiographic Region with regard vertebrate species richness.

RVhexID – Data frame of hexagon ID numbers in the Ridge & Valley Physiographic Region.

RVhexIDs – Data frame of hexagon ID numbers in the Ridge & Valley Physiographic Region.

RVhexOrd – Salient scaling on four variates for hexagons in the Ridge & Valley Physiographic Region.

RVhexOrds – Salient scaling on vertebrate species richness and percent forest cover for hexagons in the Ridge & Valley Physiographic Region.

RVhexRank – Data frame of place ranks for four variates of hexagons in the Ridge & Valley Physiographic Region.

RVhexRnk – Data frame of place ranks for vertebrate species richness of hexagons in the Ridge & Valley Physiographic Region.

RVhexs – Data frame of four variates for hexagons in the Ridge & Valley Physiographic Region.

RVhexsp – Data frame of vertebrate species richness for hexagons in the Ridge & Valley Physiographic Region.

RVpairs – Data frame of hexagon neighbors and largest open patch for hexagons in the Ridge & Valley Physiographic Region.

RVpairsp – Data frame of hexagon neighbors and percent forest for hexagons in the Ridge & Valley Physiographic Region.

Salnt11Q2Q3 – Salient scaling of 11 contingents based on product-order relation for second and third quartiles of representative ranks.

Salnt11Q1Q2Q3 – Salient scaling of 11 contingents based on product-order relation for quartiles of representative ranks.

SalntEcol – Salient sequence of ecological value and ecological sensitivity for Italian case study.

SalntEcols – Case-ordered joint salient scaling of ecological value and ecological sensitivity for Italian case study.

SalntHumn – Salient sequence of human pressure for Italian case study.

SalntHumns – Case-ordered salient scaling of human pressure for Italian case study.

SalntPCO – Data frame combining salient scalings from SalntPCO11, SalntPCO11R, and SalntPCO11S.

SalntPCO11 – Salient scaling of 11 contingents based on product-order relation for principal coordinates of centroids according to original scaling of variates.

SalntPCO11R – Salient scaling of 11 contingents based on product-order relation for principal coordinates of centroids according to place ranks of variates.

SalntPCO11S – Salient scaling of 11 contingents based on product-order relation for principal coordinates of centroids according to standardized scaling of variates.

Salnts – Data frame of salient scalings for three suites of indicators in Italian case study.

SalntSntv – Salient sequence of ecological sensitivity for Italian case study.

SalntSntvs – Case-ordered salient scaling of ecological sensitivity for Italian case study.

SalntValu – Salient sequence of ecological value for Italian case study.

SalntValus – Case-ordered salient scaling of ecological value for Italian case study.

ToppingOrd – Partial pool placements for hexagons in Toppings pool.

Toppings – Pool of selected well-placed hexagons from contingents 4, 5, 6, 7, and 10 according to salient scaling on first five variates.

ToppingAA – Aggregate advantage levels for hexagons in Toppings pool.

ToppingSS – Subordinate step levels for hexagons in Toppings pool.

TopRR – Pool of selected well-placed hexagons from contingents 4, 5, 6, 7, and 10 according to salient scaling of representative ranks for first five variates.

TopRRof4 – Selected well-placed hexagons in contingent 4 according to salient scaling of representative ranks.

TopRRof5 – Selected well-placed hexagons in contingent 5 according to salient scaling of representative ranks.

TopRRof6 – Selected well-placed hexagons in contingent 6 according to salient scaling of representative ranks.

TopRRof7 – Selected well-placed hexagons in contingent 7 according to salient scaling of representative ranks.

TopRRof10 – Selected well-placed hexagons in contingent 10 according to salient scaling of representative ranks.

TopRRord – Partial pool placements based on minimum and maximum representative ranks for hexagons in TopRR pool.

TopRRSS – Subordinate step levels based on minimum and maximum representative ranks for hexagons in TopRR pool.

TopRRSSmmm – Subordinate step levels based on minimum, median and maximum representative ranks for hexagons in TopRR pool.

TopRRAA – Aggregate advantage levels based on minimum and maximum representative ranks for hexagons in TopRR pool.

TopRRAAmmm – Aggregate advantage levels based on minimum, median and maximum representative ranks for hexagons in TopRR pool.

TopRRordmmm – Partial pool placements based on minimum, median and maximum representative ranks for hexagons in TopRR pool.

TopsOf4 – Selected well-placed hexagons in contingent 4 according to salient scaling on first five variates.

TopsOf5 – Selected well-placed hexagons in contingent 5 according to salient scaling on first five variates.

TopsOf6 – Selected well-placed hexagons in contingent 6 according to salient scaling on first five variates.

TopsOf104 – Selected well-placed hexagons in contingent 10 according to salient scaling on first five variates.

V – (In Chap. 14): Eigenvectors for canonical axis (discriminant) analysis of Groups I, II, and III.

W – (In Chap. 14): Pooled within-groups (I, II, and III) covariance matrix.

W1 – Within-group covariance matrix for hexagons in Group I (IhexS).

W2 – Within-group covariance matrix for hexagons in Group II (IIhexS).

W3 – Within-group covariance matrix for hexagons in Group III (IIIhexS).

Xbase – Basis vectors of BAMBI6 data under decorrelation (principal component) transformation as row-wise cases.

Xbasis – Basis vectors of BAMBIS data under decorrelation (principal component) transformation as row-wise cases.

Xpand – Hexagons to be annexed onto select sector of Ridge & Valley Physiographic Region.

Xpands – Hexagons to be annexed onto select sector of Ridge & Valley Physiographic Region with regard vertebrate species richness.

Index